Real Help

FOR

PLANTAR FASCIITIS

DR PETE MONCADO, DC

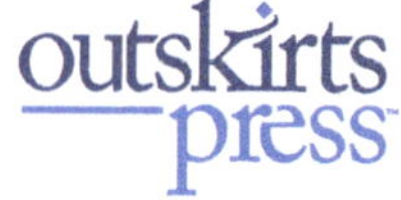

The suggestions and recommendations in this book are specific yet very generalized. Every condition is different. Consult with your physician to verify or confirm the type of condition you may have before making any assumptions. If attempting to follow any of the recommendations presented herein results in further injury, pain, or major discomfort, stop and consult your physician. Minor discomfort can be expected in some cases.

TABLE OF CONTENTS

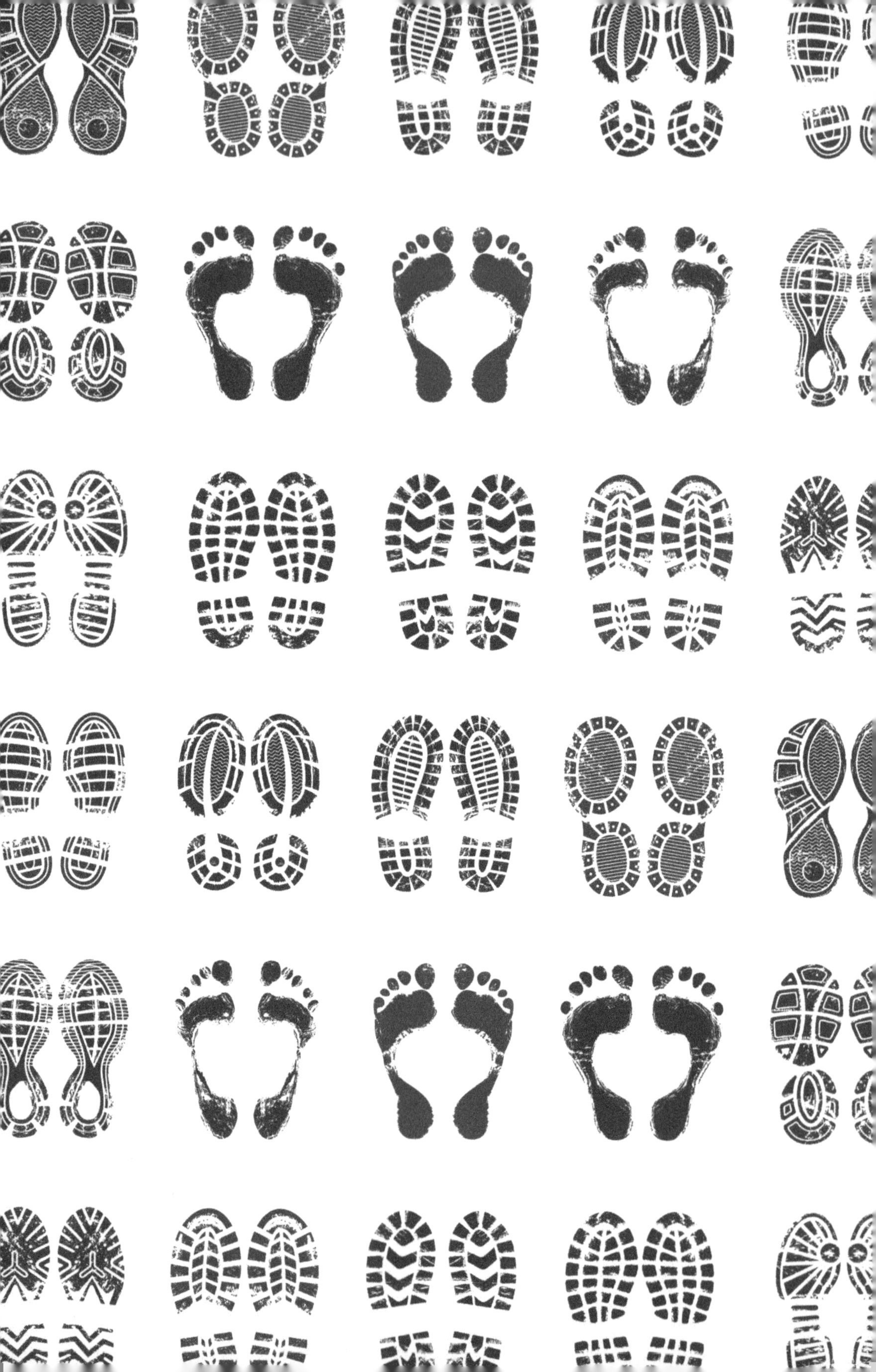

FOREWORD

God created all things. He is the giver of all life, and He made things in such a way that they exist with detailed structure and order. His greatest invention of all is **us**

Psalm 139:14 says: *I praise You because I am fearfully and wonderfully made; Your works are wonderful, I know that full well.*

The human body is truly a designed masterpiece. It has the ability to adapt to its environment, eat and digest food, heal, and regenerate itself on a cellular level every day. A simple yet profound aspect is our structural design.

Our skeletal system is made up of several bones and joints of many shapes and sizes. What's important to understand is that these bones form a very specific and unique relationship with one another in a structural relationship that affects our ability to function and move. Relative to this, our feet are one of the most important components of the entire skeletal system.

Our feet are remarkable. They are made up of several small bones that fit together like a puzzle. They are structurally designed to be both rigid and flexible, to stabilize and propel, and to hold us steady and move the rest of our body from one place to another. These functions make our feet supremely important in just about every aspect of our lives. Having healthy, happy feet allows us to live within the realm of our daily routines without the interruption of constant pain and discomfort. My hope, to which I am earnestly dedicated, is that after reading this material, the benefits to you will be tremendous.

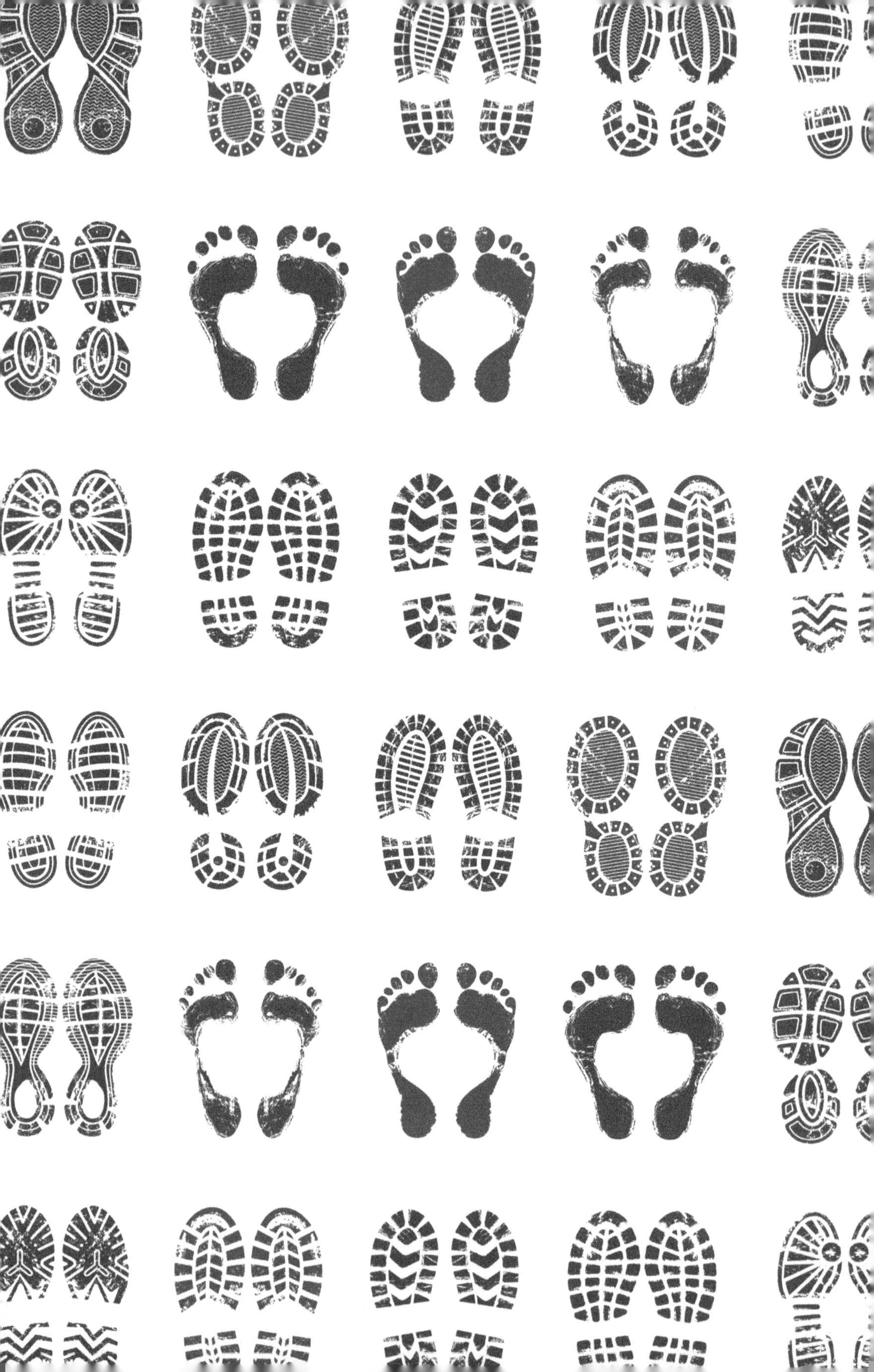

Introduction

As a chiropractic student, I was pretty excited to be learning about the human body. I had always been fascinated with physical fitness and how the body worked.

Right about the time I started my studies at chiropractic college, I was only in my twenties but already had a problem with my foot. The pain was on the bottom of my right foot, between two small bones, near the back. I was always trying to alleviate the pain through stretching or massage. Still, it bothered me constantly. In fact, I was in chronic pain.

When I reached my senior year, we had an extremities course taught by a renowned chiropractor from the Bay Area with an extremity practice. He was extremely skilled with feet.

One day, after class, I approached him to discuss my problem. He had me come into his office, where he assessed it; then, he made some adjustments on it. Wow! What an amazing difference. It freed up my foot tremendously, and I felt much better. Those adjustments allowed my foot to begin healing. The chronicity, or chronic type of pain, that I had experienced there for so long was slowly dissipating. Because of the adjustments, I was able to maintain an active lifestyle. So, I thought to myself, "Well, there's something to this," and I continued to see him as a patient.

When my own issues were resolved, and following successful treatments of my patients early in my career, the light bulb came on for me, so to speak. That was a turning point in my mind. I knew that was the direction I wanted to go. My personal experience is what spring-boarded me into the program that I'm offering now.

This program has been developed and improved through the years. It has not only been highly successful for patients with similar problems to my own but also for patients with issues far worse than mine.

Over time, I've been able to gain input from podiatrists as well. I attended the annual podiatric conference in San Diego several years ago, and it provided a tremendous wealth of information. After the conference, I knew I had something unique to offer in an area that few chiropractors focus on as their main emphasis.

My knowledge and experience opened up the door for me to help people with foot issues who had yet to find relief elsewhere. For example, I came across a gentleman who was limping his way through a health fair. He walked up to my booth, and we started chatting. I asked him what was causing his limp. He was a runner who had injured his foot and ankle on a trail in the forest. He had tried to jump over a log and landed on a rock.

Since the time of his injury, he had seen several different types of doctors and undergone several types of treatment, but nothing had worked for him. None of the doctors he'd seen had any answers. Everything they offered him was a *temporary* fix: some *temporary* steroid shots, *temporary* Band-Aids for the pain.

The results were always the same: their effectiveness would wear off, and he'd still be in pain. He had even been told, *"You just have to learn to live with it, and you won't be able to run again."* The bottom line was this: he was left feeling hopeless.

Without hesitation, I told him to come into the clinic where I would be able to find the root cause of his problem and be able to treat his injury. He did, and, within just a few months, not only was he pain-free, but he was running again! What joy it gives me to know he is living an active life again!

A few years ago, a woman who was referred to my office came hobbling in on crutches. She couldn't put weight on her foot because of an injury she had suffered while wearing high heels. She said she had endured the problem for quite some time and was desperate for help. She had tried four different podiatrists and was not getting any results. I assessed the problem and found the root cause of her pain. It took a few months, but her problem was resolved, and she was able to walk normally once again.

These are just two examples of the many types of similar cases I have been able to help through the years. I have been able to help those who felt hopeless and been able to restore health and hope to a patient's life, which is what makes it all worthwhile. The results that I've seen with my patients are exactly why I continue to develop my knowledge and work in this field.

As a chiropractor, I want to talk about the ***natural approach*** to treating plantar fasciitis, or PF. It's something I'm very passionate about, and thousands of people suffer from it daily. Most people think of chiropractors as only back and neck doctors, but interestingly enough, we can apply our skills to the feet as well. There are many different programs and a wealth of knowledge available today regarding plantar fasciitis. I am a cheerleading advocate of anything that can help someone get the relief they need.

Whether it's a book, class, or seminar, I take the "one thing" approach. If there is at least one piece of information I can apply that makes me a better practitioner or person in some way, then it is worth the effort.

Though not everything in this book may apply to every single individual who reads it, if one thing can make a beneficial impact on someone's life, then it was worth sharing this information. As you read, look for that one thing that impacts you, and then be ready for more.

So, let's begin our journey.

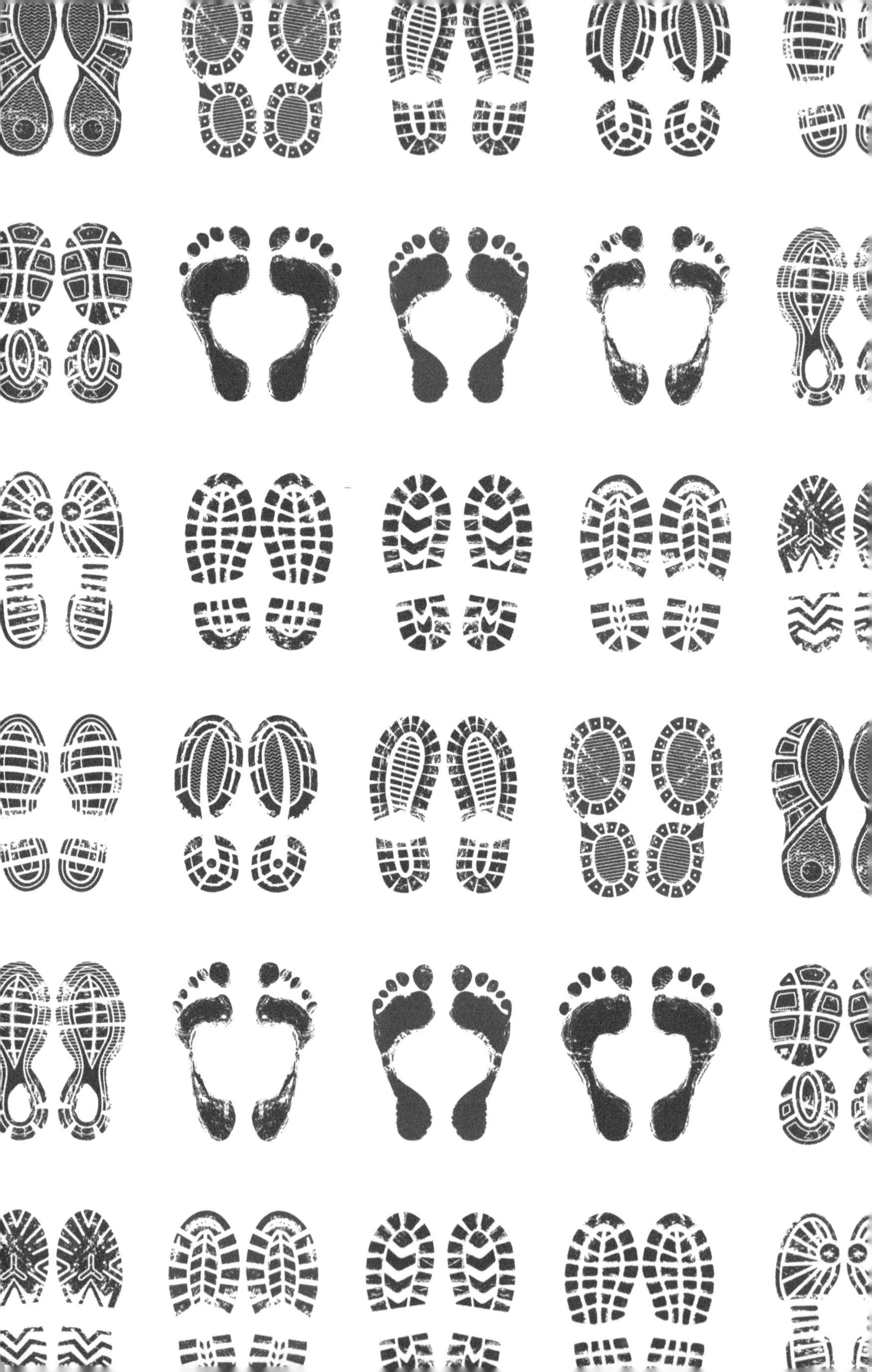

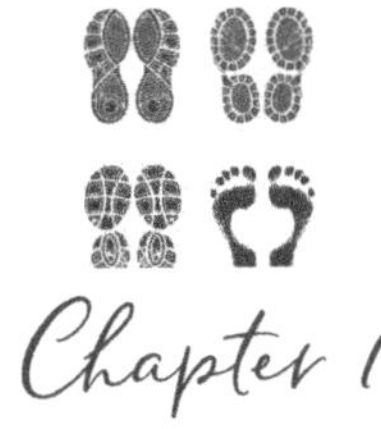

Chapter 1

AN ALTERNATIVE APPROACH

Most people think of chiropractic as bone popping or cracking that's usually only for the back, not the feet. A chiropractor is a primary care entry-level physician (yes, we are actually doctors) who specializes in correcting the joints of the skeletal system using a method called *adjustment*. An adjustment is a gentle thrust applied to a bone that is out of position to restore it to its natural position, thereby relieving injured tissue and allowing it to heal. This can be done with the hands or special adjusting instruments that have been invented for just that purpose.

A chiropractic adjustment is pressure applied directly to the bone at a **specific angle** to correct *subluxation* (misalignment) and realign the bones back to their proper joint position. This can allow for healing of the tissues and reduce inflammation.

Many times, chiropractors are called "quacks and witch doctors." However, those types of statements are made in ignorance by those who do not fully understand what the chiropractor actually does. In fact, a chiropractic education involves considerably more hours of anatomy and physiology than that of a general MD. Most of the public would not know that. Most people would also not know that chiropractic doesn't involve just the neck and back; in fact, chiropractic can also help the feet.

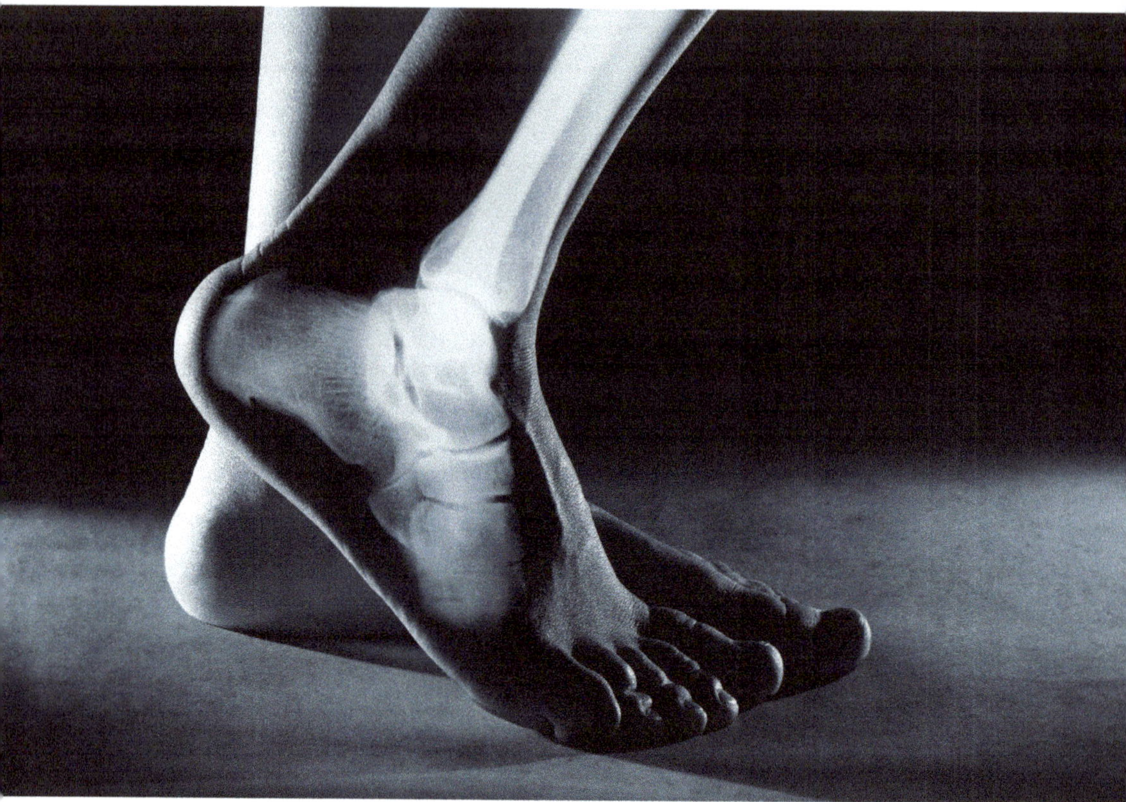

Healthy, happy feet aren't just pain-free; they also work properly. We should have the ability to get around without struggling or dealing with limitations on what we can or cannot do. Those of us who have experienced chronic foot pain know that this can be very frustrating, especially for athletes.

It can be frustrating not only for professional athletes but for weekend warriors too: those of us who engage in pick-up sports, who exercise at the gym, hike the trails, and pound the pavement. We all want to be able to do these things comfortably and with ease.

For those of us who are nonprofessional athletes, running and jogging are among the most popular forms of exercise worldwide. We want to be able to move freely on our feet without any hindrance. It's essential to performance as well as peace of mind. Many times, in the athletic world, injuries go unresolved.

The ability to live a normal everyday life and carry out routines without having to stop and sit down due to the pain in our feet should be and can become a standard for nearly everyone. Having healthy, happy feet is what we all want, and it should be a part of our daily lives.

By properly addressing the mechanical deficiencies of plantar fasciitis first, and in a very specific way, is where we begin the process of treatment. When accumulative damage has occurred to the point that surgery is required, we are faced with an extremely significant problem. Do you think we were born into this world requiring metal plates in our feet simply to walk? Under normal circumstances, absolutely not. So, what if that type of situation can be prevented? The techniques I've learned do exactly that: they help people avoid ever reaching that level. It's so gratifying to help people become empowered in such a way that they can take some control of their own body, their own health, their own feet—not only to heal but also to *prevent* plantar fasciitis, or PF.

Preventing injuries before they actually happen is one of the best ways to avoid the misery that PF and related foot issues can cause. Any injury, discomfort, or pain always has a *root* cause. In order for any ailment to be resolved, we must find out what that is. Finding the actual cause allows the body to begin the healing process.

A standard and common treatment for plantar fasciitis is corticosteroids in the form of injections. This is more or less a *Band-Aid* approach because it eases the pain until the shots wear off—but then what? We, as a culture, want instant gratification, but that just isn't how the body works.

What about the mechanical portion of the foot injury? Did the shots resolve that portion of it? Not at all. Many patients fall for the trap that an injection, a pill, or a muscle relaxant will fix the problem. However, the effect of the medication is quite often only temporary. This is why many of these cases still go unresolved. We often see commercials about a quick fix or medications that will make specific health problems go away instantly, but that just isn't so when it comes to chronic PF.

Regardless of the health issue involved, it has to go through the process of **healing** to actually get better. Healing an injury is never instant unless it's Divine—in the category of a miracle. Our bodies need time to heal. For instance, if you broke your arm, what's the first thing you'd have done to treat it? You'd have a cast put on. Why a cast? To keep it protected and stable while it **heals.** Does it heal the next day? Of course not. In the same way, we want to learn how to allow our bodies to become the ultimate healing machine from the inside out. We do that by learning what things are good for our bodies and what things aren't.

I was watching tv one night, and a commercial came on about a medication. In the commercial, it showed happy smiling people riding bicycles and doing family-type things. Very healthy, happy, and laughing and smiling. However, toward the end of it, they started to list several side effects. The people in the commercial were still smiling… There were many effects listed, but the one that stood out the most was that it could possibly cause sudden death. Really?!?!

Sudden death!! Hmm…that one sounds like a real winner for well-being and peace of mind!

The point is, when we blindly rely on external synthetic substances for just about any pain or issue we have, we are potentially robbing ourselves of the greatest medicine cabinet of all: **ourselves.** God made our bodies with the ability to heal **naturally**. As we journey through this book, my hope is to pass some knowledge on to you while inspiring habits conducive to your well-being.

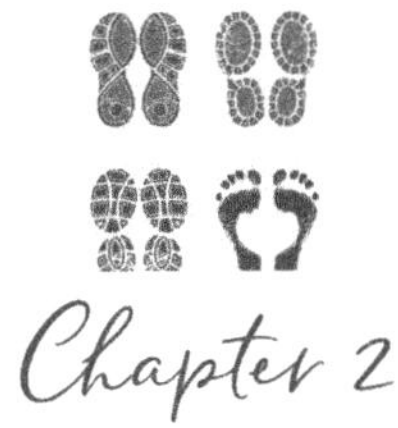

Chapter 2

UNDERSTANDING WHAT PLANTAR FASCIITIS REALLY IS

The simplest way to explain plantar fasciitis is that it is simply a symptom, not a cause. The *plantar fascia* is a fibrous ligamentous tissue that runs from the heel, across the bottom of the foot, extending to the big toe. If there are underlying structural problems with an individual's feet, it can cause the fascia to become damaged microscopically. This results in the common condition known as *plantar fasciitis*. Simply put, plantar fasciitis is an injury to the plantar fascia, causing it to become inflamed and irritated.

The suffix *-itis* means **inflamed.** Any ailment with the suffix *-itis* attached means it's an inflammatory condition. Inflammation can be caused by many different things, but the one characteristic, regardless of the cause, is *"**It hurts!**"*

There are approximately two million Americans per year who seek some type of medical or pain relief treatment for plantar fasciitis. This indicates that it is quite prevalent. The question is, *why*? What's the cause of this debilitating, unpleasant condition? The answers are found by looking at the underlying causes of tissue inflammation. Thus, in the feet, we want to start by looking at the *structure*. This means addressing the mechanical portion of the foot.

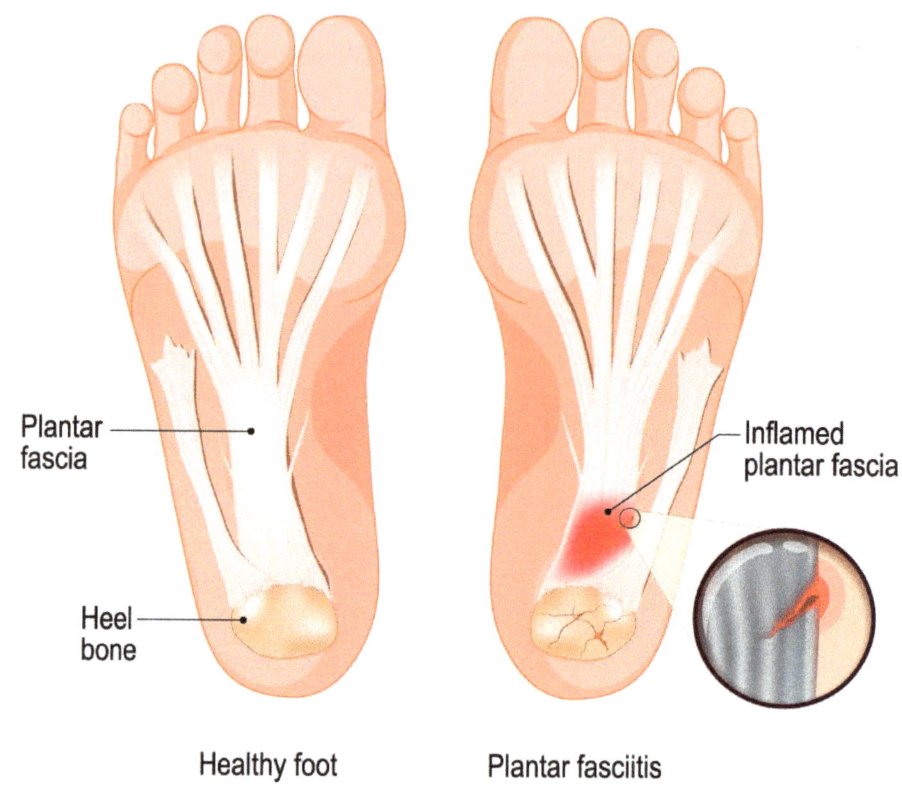

There are generally two components involved in PF: *inflammatory* and ***mechanical*** (structural). Here's the key to understanding the process of repair regarding the treatment of PF:

The mechanical issue usually comes first, not the inflammatory. In most of our PF cases, only the inflammatory portion has been dealt with, not the structural. This leaves the mechanical issue unresolved. Steroid injections can last up to three months on average; however, once these wear off, the pain can return, and the mechanical issue is still there. This treatment cycle will often continue to repeat as the underlying mechanical issue worsens over time. At that point, even pain-relieving medication has very little to no effect.

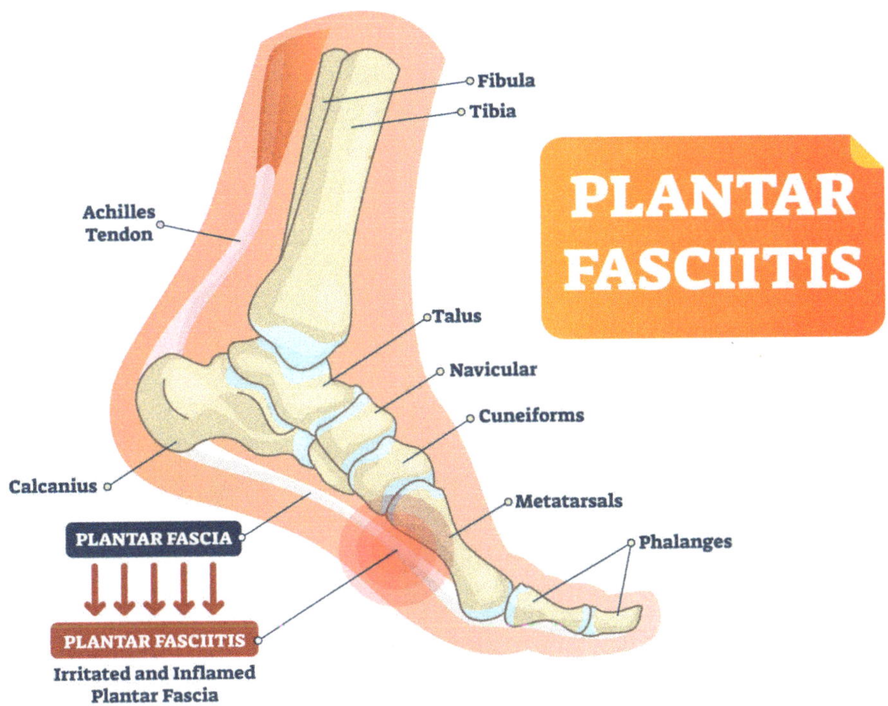

The key to solving any plantar fasciitis case is finding the actual cause, not the symptom.

PLANTAR FASCIITIS

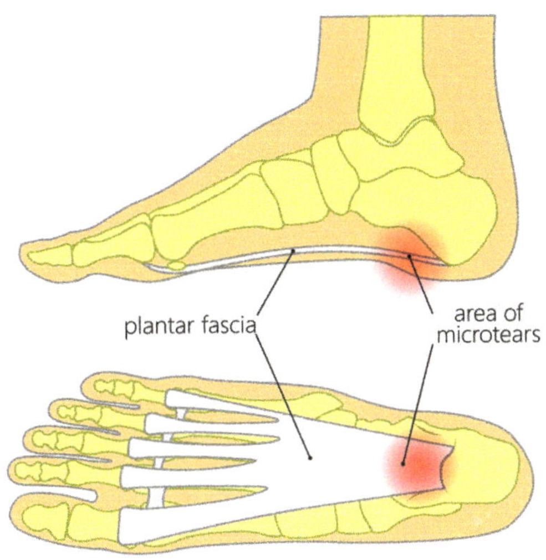

Pain is the symptom, but what caused that pain to begin with? As mentioned earlier, our feet are structurally designed to support our body weight and move us from one place to another. They are *mechanical* in nature, and their structure is very important to how well they function. Plantar fasciitis involves three components of our anatomy that need to be addressed:

Muscles
Connective tissue
Bones/joints

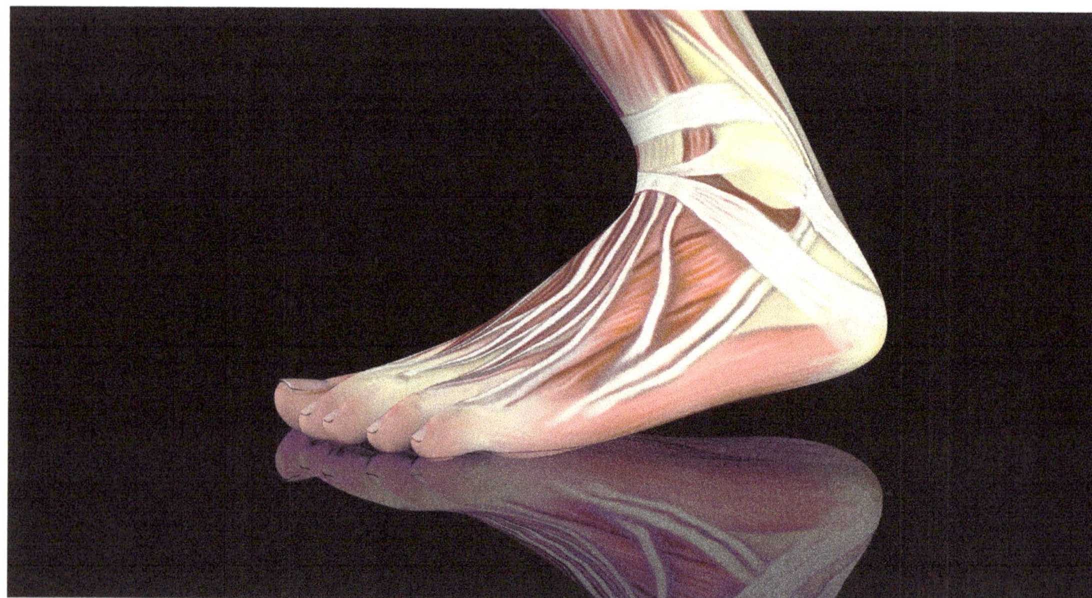

These three components of our feet and ankles need to be working together harmoniously in order for everything to eventually get better. It is here where we will start our assessment. If any one of these areas is compromised, it won't be long before the other two will follow.

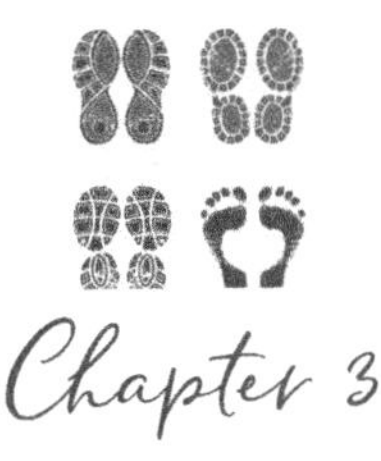

Chapter 3
WHAT HAPPENS IF
WE WAIT TOO LONG?

What happens if we only treat our pain with painkillers and medications and not the actual cause? If we just mask the symptoms temporarily? Think of it like this: let's say you break your arm. The initial pain lasts for days. As a result, you take pain killers, and they actually work terrifically to the point that your arm feels great. It feels so good, in fact, that you decide you want to go out and do yard work and gardening. It's a beautiful sunny day. You go about it enjoying yourself, smelling the fresh air and flowers. You feel wonderful! No arm pain. ***But the fracture is still there.*** You go about shoveling and digging with no pain—they were very strong painkillers. However, they eventually wear off. By nightfall, the pain in your arm from the fracture is excruciating. You can't even move it. Why??

Not only was the initial cause of the pain still very much present in your arm (the fracture), but you damaged it further by masking that pain and using your arm when you shouldn't have. In a similar way, we can't just stop walking. We can't stop living our everyday lives. If we mask our PF pain and symptoms and do not treat the cause, we are doing the same thing as in the previous scenario.

The bottom line is this: continuing to ignore or not to have the root cause properly addressed can lead to secondary conditions that can be even more serious than the plantar fasciitis symptoms. Listed below are seven of the most common problems

1. Heel spurs/heel pain

Ignoring heel pain can have potentially catastrophic consequences for your feet. Heel pain is the most common area of pain in PF patients. The plantar fascia connects to the inner part of the heel bone (calcaneus), and its surrounding tissues are continually stressed over time by the altered foot mechanics. This causes calcium deposits and a growth that protrudes from the calcaneus called a *heel spur*. These can be extremely painful.

2. Arthritis

Degenerative arthritis is something that occurs in joints due to stressful wear and tear on the tissues surrounding the joints. This can lead to the disintegration of cartilage and the fusion of bones. When bones fuse together, it's as if they become one clumped bone. This would be considered a form of permanent damage in the sense that the joint is basically replaced by bone and calcification.

3. Bunions

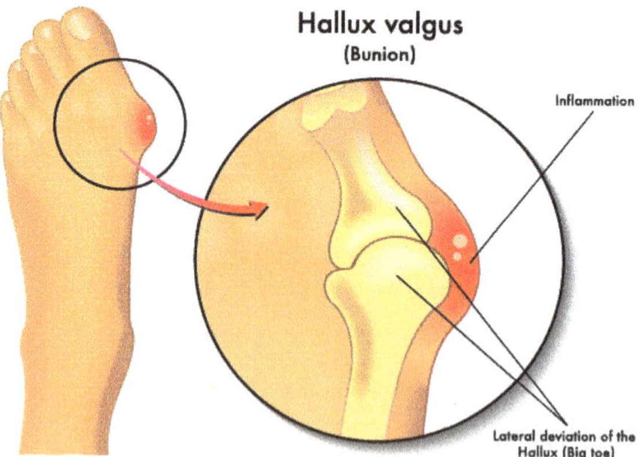

Bunions can form when something causes the first joint of the big toe to go out of alignment. When other foot bones misalign, this can cause the first joint of the big toe to follow. Over a period of time, walking with abnormal pressure on it causes a bunion to form. Women who wear high heels are at a higher risk. Bunion formation can be slowed by correcting structural issues in the foot, but they can only be removed surgically. Thus, if mechanical problems are fixed early on, the potential for bunions to occur is much less.

4. Knee pain

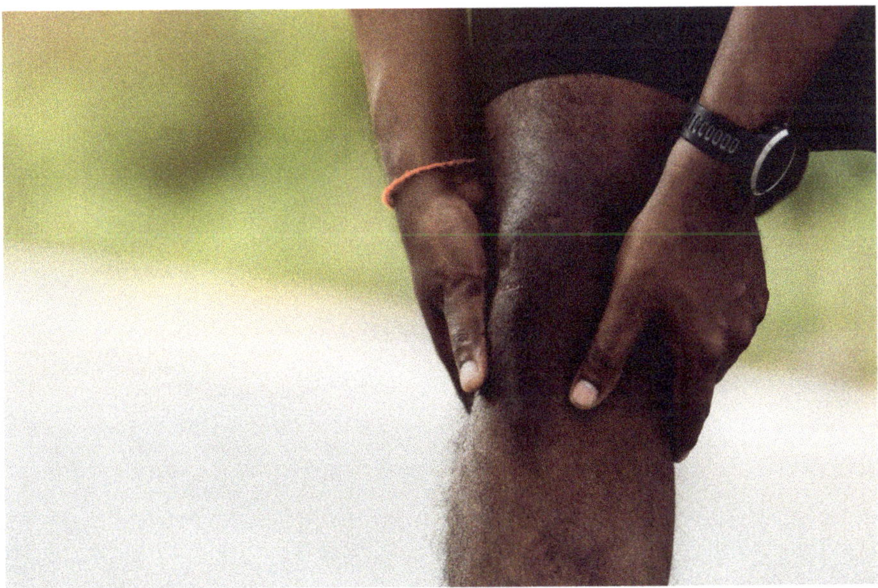

When the feet aren't working right mechanically, it puts tremendous stress on our knees. Remember, our feet are like shock absorbers; if force or pressure isn't being absorbed properly by our feet, this can put heavy strain on the knees, leading to potential issues such as tendinitis, bursitis, or osteoarthritis.

5. Back Pain

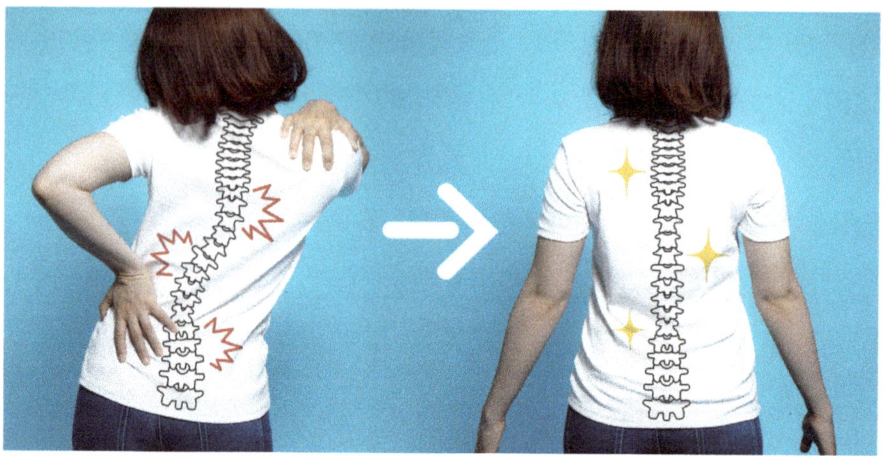

Our feet affect our alignment. Walking in a way that exerts abnormal pressure (with a slight limp or placing more pressure on one foot) can cause our spine and hips to misalign. This can lead to back pain and discomfort over time. Having our feet corrected helps to align our posture.

6. Risk of Achilles tendon strain or tear

If we don't have full use of the natural shock-absorbing ability of our feet, and we are exerting heavy loads of force on them, i.e., during athletic events or running, we put ourselves at risk of injuring tendons and ligaments further up the leg. A severe tear or rupture of the Achilles tendon requires surgical repair.

7. Compensatory foot pain

In all my years of practice, I have yet to find a single plantar fasciitis case in which both feet hurt exactly the same. Usually, one foot hurts worse than the other. What can happen if the patient continues to walk in such a state? The uninjured foot can develop problems from overcompensating for the more injured foot. Treating the condition early on helps to alleviate further development of plantar fasciitis in both feet.

The first signs that alert us to an injured foot tend to be obvious. There's going to be discomfort and pain. It's painful to take a step, especially in the morning. The pain can develop suddenly or over time without an actual accident or traumatic event; so, what happened? The bottom line is this: there was a breakdown in the structure somehow in one or more of the following: the bones, joints, connective tissue, or muscles.

It is critical to understand that to resolve our foot issues thoroughly, we have to look beyond just the pain. The underlying problems that caused the pain in the first place must be adequately dealt with to get the desired results. Just one underlying root cause of untreated plantar fasciitis can lead to a cascade of many secondary problems discussed earlier in this chapter. Thus, it is imperative to take the right approach sooner than later.

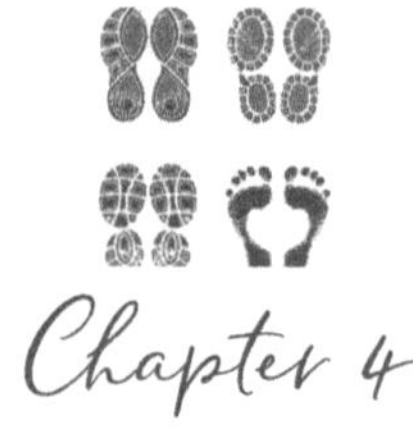

THINGS WE DO TO INITIATE PLANTAR FASCIITIS

What activities or other things in our lives can potentially cause structural issues that lead to PF?

Listed below are five of what I have found in my clinical experience to be the most common causes:

Improper footwear

Poor footwear is the most common factor that can cause havoc to our feet. Wearing improper shoes, over time, can do significant damage, sometimes beyond repair. Developing proper foot health from the time we are toddlers to adulthood is vital. It is in these developmental stages of life that our feet can be greatly affected, along with the knees, ankles, hips and spine. This means that getting the proper shoes and fit is of vital importance the moment we put on our very first pair.

Improper footwear can cause the bones of the feet to shift out of their normal joint position slowly. These misalignments then cause the muscles, ligaments, and tendons to become weak. Our feet become deformed and eventually injured as they weaken, leading to pain and discomfort. Chapter 10 will cover footwear in more detail.

Trauma

Injuries during accidents, sports injuries, or repetition.

Improperly placed arch supports

The improper placement of shoe supports can cause significant stress to our feet. This, in turn, leads to tissue irritation and joint discomfort. It can also lead to the joints in the feet becoming slightly displaced. Thus, it is critical to have properly fitting foot supports to avoid repetitive foot injuries by careful placement and proper fit.

High impact sports

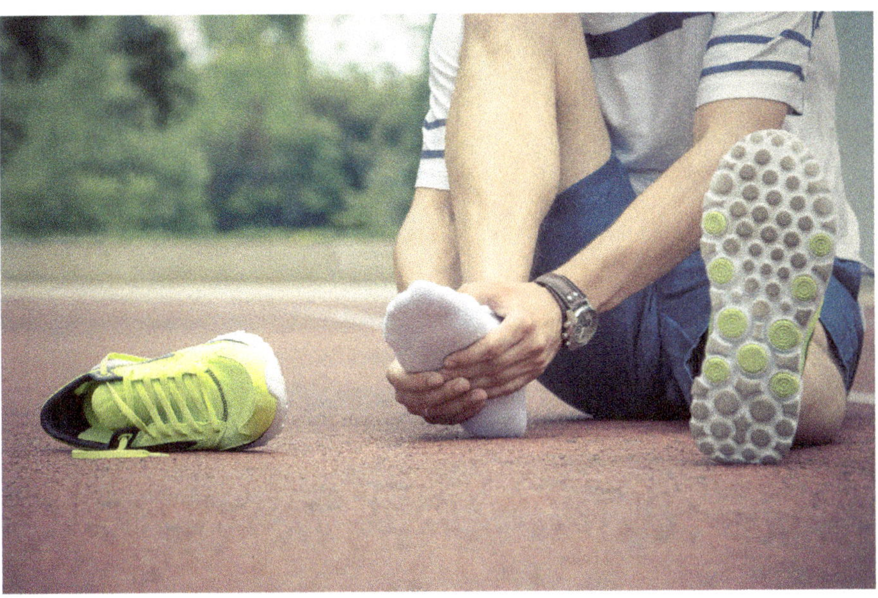

Running or jogging can exert three times your body weight in impact force per step: doing this repeatedly can cause stress fractures, misalignments, and other injuries.

As the joints, muscles, and tendons in our feet become weak or altered, bones can shift slightly out of their normal position. This condition has a special name. It's called **subluxation** (pronounced sub-lux-AY-shun).

Think of it like this: If a bone shifts way out of its joint position to the point of being detached, it's called a *dislocation*. If it's only slightly out of position and not fully detached, this is called a subluxation. This condition will be further explained in the treatment section.

Subluxations can cause microscopic tearing of connective tissues and muscle tightness. In many cases, prolonged daily stress on the feet due to improper footwear and subluxation, causes underlying structural issues that produce tearing and inflammation, leading to pain and discomfort.

Wear and tear and repetitive pressure on structurally compromised feet can be a major factor in developing plantar fasciitis. The fascia can **re-tear over and over** just from everyday walking, stretching, or certain other activities. Sometimes this can happen when individuals are trying to resolve PF on their own.

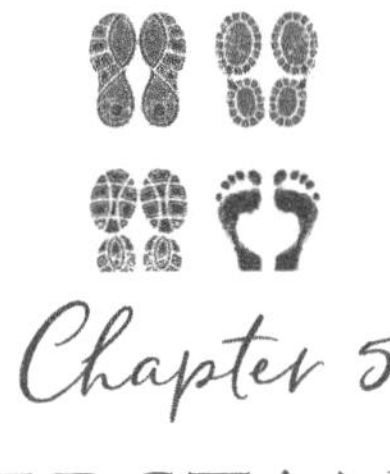

Chapter 5
UNDERSTANDING NORMAL VS ABNORMAL

As is always the case, before we can ever truly define abnormal, we must first be able to define normal.

A normal human foot (structurally and anatomically) consists of 26 bones and 33 joints and has over 100 muscles and tendons. Its overall shape and structure reflect its functional design (Wikipedia).

Our feet are naturally adaptive. They have the ability to be strong and rigid and yet flexible and relaxed when needed.

Looking at the diagram, we see bones of different shapes and sizes, among which are cuboidal or rectangular. These bones are designed to align and connect with each other in very specific ways.

Foot anatomy
(bones of the foot)

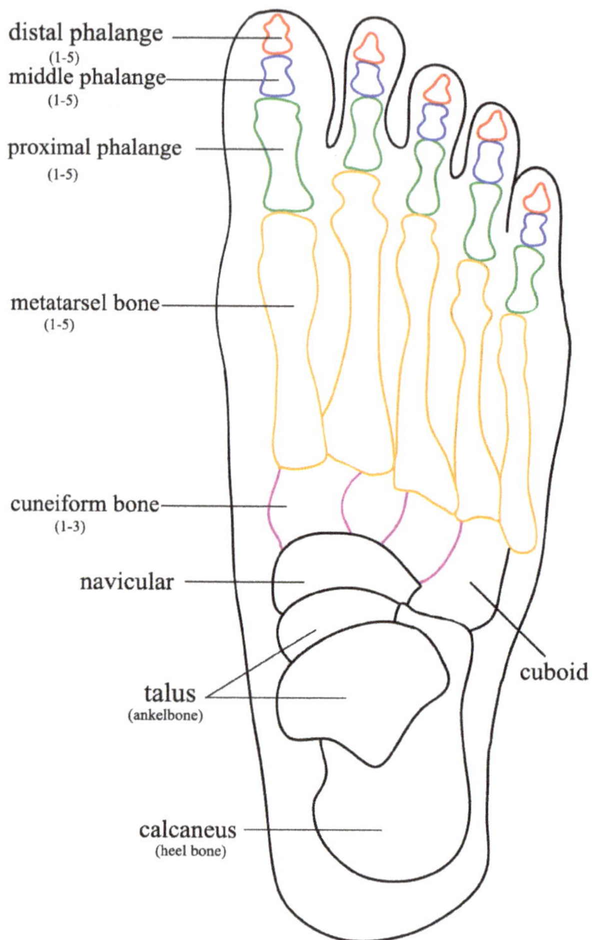

Tarsal bones are near the rear part of our feet. These consist of the **talus, calcaneus, navicular, cuboid,** and the **cuneiforms.** They all connect in a way that is designed for optimal foot function and biomechanics.

Looking at the foot from the side, on the inside part of the foot, we see there's an arch in the middle of the foot. The position of the bones relative to one another plays a factor in forming a normal arch. If these bones become positionally compromised, the arch can become collapsed or elevated, either too little or too much. Bones in the feet shifting ***ever so slightly*** can have huge ramifications.

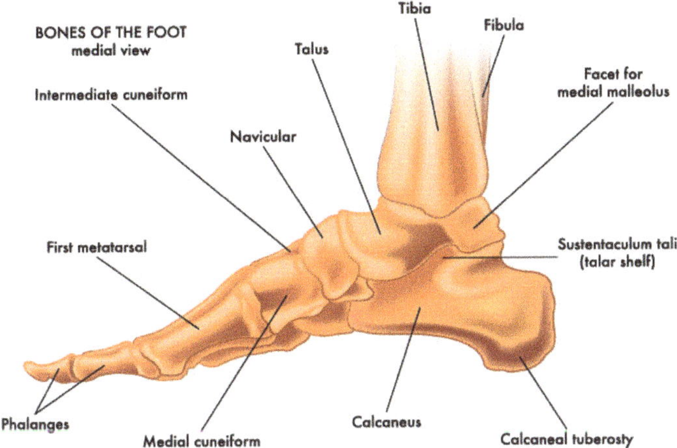

Even a normal foot can still develop pain from fatigue from prolonged overuse. Standing at work all day is a good example of that. However, structural issues, such as flat feet and high-arched feet, are not considered normal. The everyday pressures of daily foot routines on these particular deformities can be cumulatively harmful, especially to the plantar fascia.

How are general foot deformities identified?

When identifying the root cause of biomechanical or structural issues in the feet, one of the first steps we can take is a ***general structural visualization.*** This is where we take a look at the three basic overall types of feet:

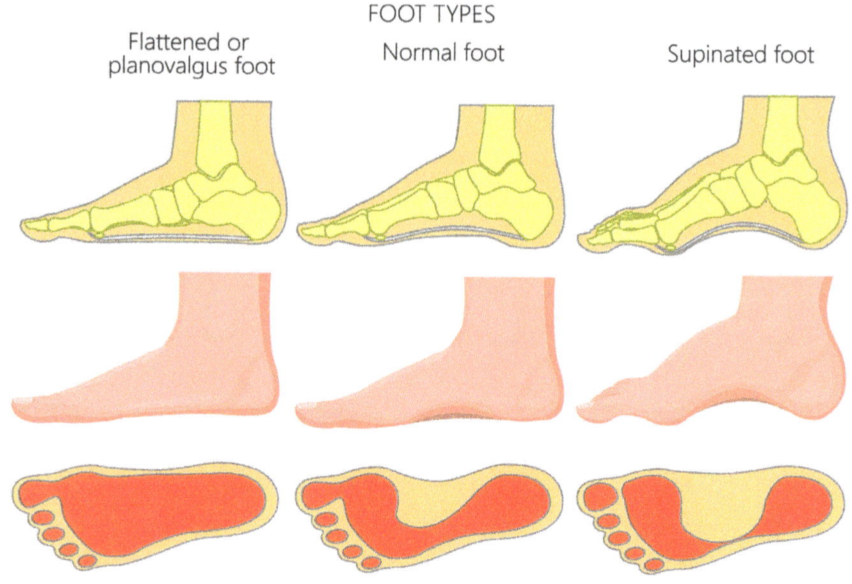

Flat feet
Normal feet
High-arched feet

These three types can have variations to differing degrees; however, normal feet generally won't have structural issues that are visible or palpable, whereas the other two will.

The greater the deformation and altered structure, the greater the risk of getting plantar fasciitis and/or secondary conditions, such a bunions.

Deformation of the foot

Flat foot (Fallen arch)			
Normal foot			
Hollow foot (High arch)			

Dropped arch/Flat feet

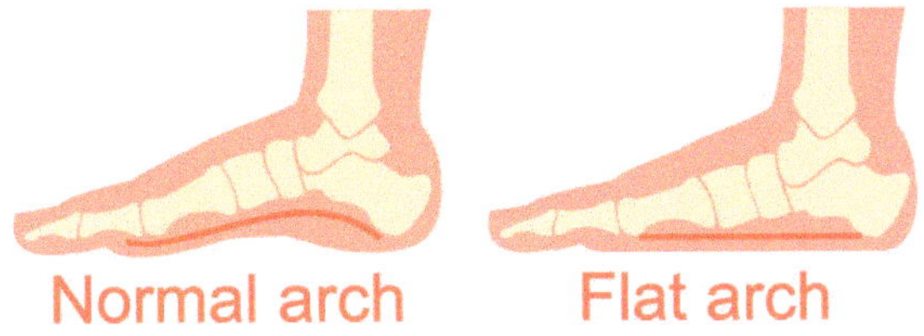

Some individuals have a collapsed arch. This is also known as a *flat foot*. This is usually associated with **pronation,** or an *inward* turning of the ankle and foot. This type of foot can oftentimes develop bunions and is frequently associated with plantar fasciitis.

The tarsal bones involved with this deformity are the ***talus***, ***navicular*** and ***medial cuneiform*** bones. These three small bones are part of the foot's inner arch (just above and in front of the heel). In a flat-footed individual, these bones are "collapsed" or "dropped down," flattening the arch. Flat arches can cause excess pressure on the tissues surrounding this area leading to potential injury. It also leads to a poor gait cycle, which can cause further problems throughout the entire foot.

High-arched/cavus foot

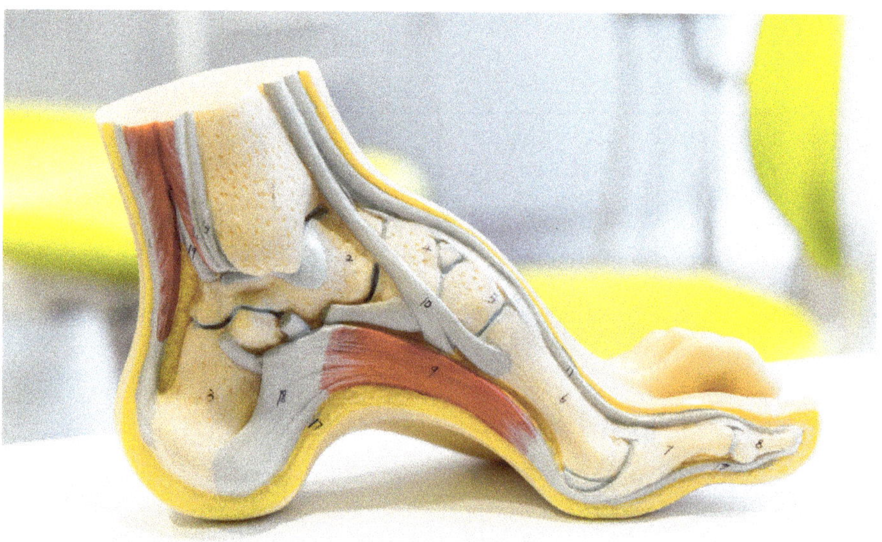

high-arched foot tends to be associated with ***supination*** (an *outward* turning of the ankle and foot). These types of deformities create abnormal foot mechanics and put great stress on the heels and balls of the feet. Also, they can cause calluses on the bottom of the foot. High-arched, or *cavus* foot, can also be associated with plantar fasciitis.

The foot bones most involved with this deformity are the ***cuboid, cuneiforms*** and ***metatarsals***. The cuboid is located at the outside of the foot just in front of the heel. It usually drops down out of alignment while the three cuneiforms, which are located to the inner side of the cuboid, are elevated upward. Because these four bones line up to form a connected "bridge" across the midfoot, the altered position gives the appearance of an "elevated" arch. The middle cuneiform often gets "sandwiched" and pushed up the furthest, between the lateral and medial cuneiform. The metatarsals (just in front of the toes) are dropped downward. As a result, tremendous pressure is placed on the forefoot and heel during walking, running, or just standing in comparison to the normal foot. When calluses are formed, they usually occur on the forefoot.

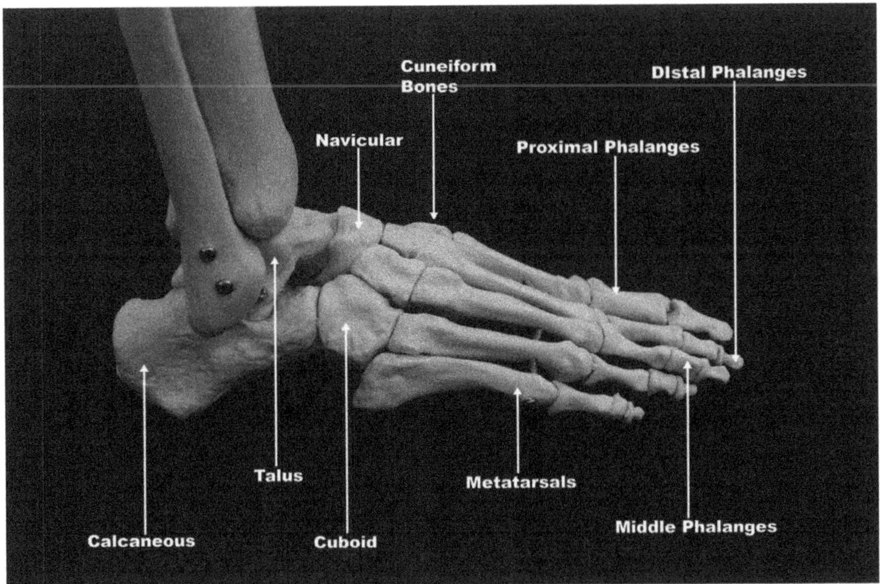

Identifying the foot type and any associated deformities is crucial to providing the proper treatment plan. Accurate identification through detailed assessment helps to implement protocols that are specific to the kind of problem presented. Chiropractic adjustments, therapies, orthotics, footwear, and shoe supports can vary depending on the type of foot and its issues. Thus, understanding the content of this chapter is of utmost importance.

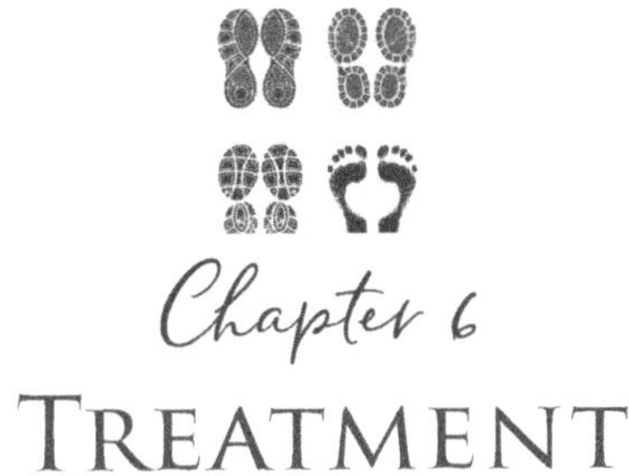

Chapter 6

TREATMENT

When our bodies are working and functioning properly, we don't just have an absence of pain: we have what is, and should be considered, normal function inside as well as out. We have **physiological balance.** Our bodies are designed to function normally in all areas.

Our bodies functioning optimally in all categories of physiology is key to healing. Injuries cannot heal in a timely manner if an individual's general health habits are poor.

Hydration

In a 2018 survey, nearly 80% of working Americans said they do not drink enough water. Our bodies are made up of mostly water (up to 60% on average). Hydration is fundamental to our overall health. In order for our bodies to heal properly, we must consider proper hydration.

It's important in flushing toxins out of our bodies. In regard to joint surfaces and bones, it's a vital component in allowing joint cushioning and flexibility of joints. Most cartilage is made of water-holding connective tissue.

An average of three liters a day of water is recommended. Of course, individual lifestyles determine whether more is needed; athletes or physical laborers and anyone who sweats more than average should drink more water.

Hydrating first thing in the morning is key to setting the body's hydration levels. *We lose water just from breathing!* Sleeping 6-8 hours without water intake means we start our day slightly below what our body actually needs.

Many times, we wake and eat first, and if it is a high carb meal (cereal, muffins, donuts, etc.), since we are already dehydrated from sleeping, this can trick our brains into thinking we are hungry when what we actually need to do is hydrate.

Try this first: when you're hungry, drink water first! Not only will it rehydrate you, but it will keep you from eating excessively. This is a simple yet great and effective approach for weight loss or maintaining body weight.

Vitamin C

Connective tissue forms **ligaments** and **tendons**. These are bands that hold our bones in place and attach muscles to them. **Cartilage** is a connective tissue that is in between bones. Because the feet contain a significant amount of connective tissue, specific nutrients are substantial to keep them healthy and robust, and one such nutrient is vitamin C.

Vitamin C is essential to these structures because it is required to make a protein called *collagen*. Collagen is a fibrous-like protein that gives ligaments, tendons, and cartilage its strength.

Without vitamin C, the body cannot make collagen. Because vitamin C is a *water-soluble* vitamin, it is not stored in the body. Thus, it must be adequately consumed through diet or supplementation.

Diet

This is a very broad topic and an entire book on its own. There are many factors that determine what to eat or not to eat. Things like lifestyle, age, level of activity, overall health, and blood type are just some of them.

There is a wealth of information out there on this topic, and my recommendation is to both consult with your physician, as well as do your own due diligence in researching what works best for you.

Relative to PF and overall health, the most important things to consider include the following:

Eating foods that are precursors for inflammation should be avoided.

Whole grains contain things that can make a substance called ***arachidonic acid.*** (Even the name sounds ominous!) This substance plays a key role in the inflammatory process. Even though whole grains can be a great source of fiber, they should be consumed carefully when the body is highly inflamed. Instead, fruit & vegetables provide a significant amount of fiber, antioxidants, and micronutrients, which benefit overall health and reduce inflammation.

High sugar/high processed carb diets in sedentary lifestyles generally lead to other potential issues such as type-2 diabetes and weight gain. These conditions can play a major role in causing greater inflammation, as well as poor overall health.

Eating to make your body less acidic

Avoiding the intake of substances that make the body more acidic will always be helpful. PH is key—the higher, the better. Many companies make alkaline water, which is designed to make your body less acidic. Eating greens and juicing raw fruits & vegetables can benefit the body's PH. Frequent juicing can provide numerous health benefits. It can also help speed up the healing process. Coffee is acidic, and intake should be limited when treating injured tissue.

Wheatgrass juice

Wheatgrass juice is considered a *"super food."* It provides tremendous benefits. It cleanses the blood and liver of toxins, and has been shown to be a powerful antioxidant. *One ounce contains the nutrients of several pounds of green vegetables.*

It has several other benefits, and this is something worth looking into. Check first to make sure you are not allergic. If not, wheatgrass juice can be of tremendous benefit to your overall health.

Eating to build a healthy immune system

Approximately 70% of our immune system is in our gut.

Different foods can build a strong immune system. Some examples are turmeric, garlic, and various herbs and mushrooms.

Along with fruits and vegetables, certain vitamins and minerals, such as zinc, vitamin C, and vitamin D are all powerful immune boosters.

Vitamin C plays a significant role in boosting immunity. It increases the formation of crucial white blood cells to help fight pathogens. It has also been beneficial in some cancer treatments.

Zinc, which is very important for the immune system, is found in red meats and nuts. It can help stop viral replication (which is a really good thing to know).

Vitamin D is very beneficial to the immune system, as well as our bone health. It can be mostly found in fortified foods and salmon. However, it can also be formed from the sun. Exposure to sunlight causes the body to change cholesterol in the blood to vitamin D. Now that is a great exchange!

Exercise

High-impact exercises should be avoided. Low impact cardio is always good as long as it doesn't overstress the joints. Swimming and cycling are good choices because they don't involve heavy ground force.

As we age, our body's flexibility lessens. Many injuries to our joints can occur when we are too tight and stiff, so stretching is important when we try to work out or exercise. If done properly, stretching can be a workout in itself.

Using proper biomechanics in all forms of stretching and exercise is of utmost importance.

Yoga and ***Tai Chi*** have been shown to be tremendous for improving flexibility and strength. The movements are generally gentle on the joints, which reduces the risk of further injury.

Posture

Most people think of good posture as "not slouching forward while standing or sitting, keeping their shoulders back, and standing as straight as possible, but that is *not* the definition of posture.

Posture, in its purest sense, is defined as the relationship of the head to the thorax (rib cage) to the pelvis.

How these three structures in your skeleton relate to one another determines your actual posture, whether good or bad.

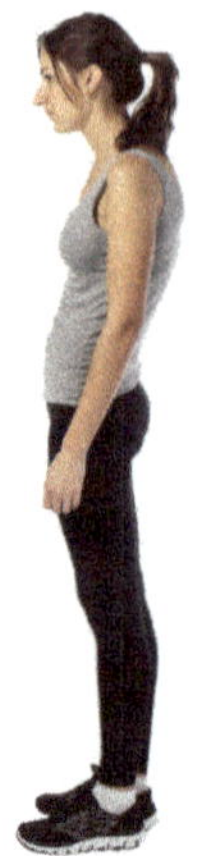 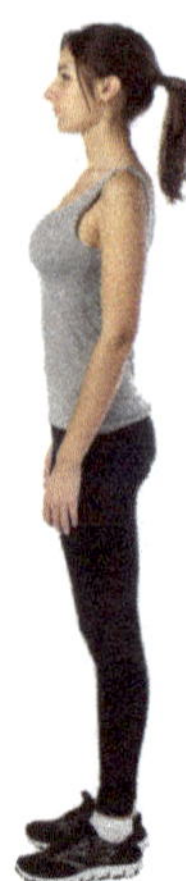

Why is posture important for overall health and in avoiding or mitigating PF?

Our structure dictates how our muscles function under the force of gravity.

Example: if our head is several inches forward, relative to the rest of our skeleton, the muscles at the base of our neck and top of our shoulders become tight and stressed. Why? Because the position of the head has shifted away from our body's center of gravity, causing these muscles to work extra hard to keep the head upright. It's as if, in theory, our head now weighs more. This can have knock-on effects, creating muscle imbalance over time.

Poor posture stresses our joints

When the force of gravity stresses our joints, the resulting adverse pressure can create wear and tear on them.

Think of it like this: if the wheels of your car are out of alignment, the tires wear down faster because they aren't centered to ensure even wear.

In the same way, if our posture is off-center, many of our joints will be as well; just going through our daily routines, in poor alignment, can cause wear and tear on our joints. For example, sitting at a computer for long hours can cause the joints, neck, and shoulders to become stressed. Just like our joints, our nerves can also become stressed. What can happen from here is ligaments and other connective tissues can become deformed.

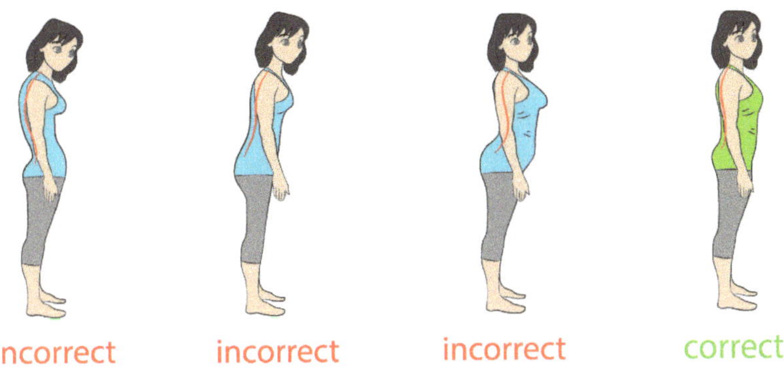

This can create slouching and a head-forward posture. When this happens, it is much more difficult to restore normal posture.

Poor posture can stress the nerves

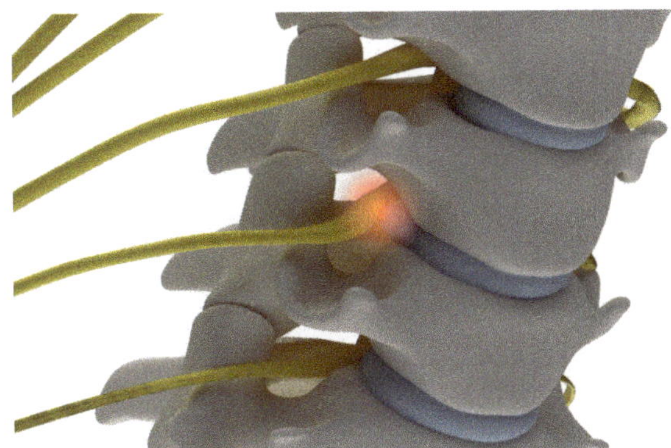

Our spinal cord is inside the bones of our spine. From there, the nerves branch out to the rest of our body. Nerve tissue is delicate and cannot withstand constant pressure. Because nerves control the whole body, they can have a crucial effect on how well our bodies function overall. Correcting misalignments in the spine can have an especially positive effect on our nervous system. In turn, it can positively affect our overall health.

Earlier, we briefly discussed **subluxation**. A subluxation is a very small displacement between two or more bones that's smaller than a dislocation. It can be so small that it's not always visible on an X-ray. It's not always something that is visible externally, either. However, it can usually be *felt* because one of the components of subluxation is a locked or jammed (fixated) joint.

A trained chiropractor is able to feel very slight displacements—even the slightest displacement—and fixations between joints and bones.

Nerve tissue is so delicate that even slight displacements can have an adverse effect on nerve tissue, especially in the spine.

This is why posture and proper spinal hygiene can play a major role in our overall health.

Alignment starts in the feet

If our feet are out of alignment, the rest of us will follow. Poor foot alignment can cause the entire body to become imbalanced as we misplace the force of impact during walking or running from our feet to the rest of our body.

Sleep

Trying to get the right amount of sleep is very important. Our bodies repair themselves and heal while we sleep. If we are not resting and sleeping, we cannot recover as quickly. Six to eight hours is optimal, but this might need to be more if an individual is sick or injured. When we sleep, we naturally release **HCG (human growth hormone)**. This hormone is very important in the rebuilding and repair of our tissues.

Being able to release this hormone and other necessary substances naturally while we sleep plays an important role in our healing.

If my patients suffer from insomnia, I usually recommend calcium before they go to bed. Calcium is a natural muscle relaxant and can help slow things down internally.

Peace of mind vs stress

Stress has been shown to be one of the top causes of health issues. Mental and emotional stress can have adverse effects on our bodies, especially if prolonged. Finding healthy outlets to release work-related stress or stress from other causes can be very helpful. Exercise, meditation, hobbies, and time in nature are just some examples.

Tai Chi and **Yoga** are very beneficial to the mind and body, as is ***Chi Gong breathing.*** These activities, and others, can be very helpful physically and mentally and are not stressful on the joints. There are many books and YouTube videos that can teach you these techniques. Find what works best for you. For me personally, having a relationship with my Lord and Savior Jesus Christ gives me, overall, the greatest peace of mind that I have ever had.

Jesus said: ***Come to me, all of you who are weary and burdened, and I will give you rest. - Matthew 11:28***

His words will never fail!

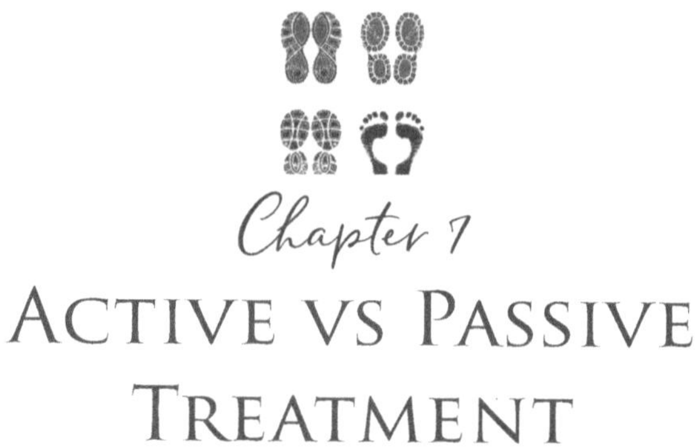

Chapter 7
ACTIVE VS PASSIVE TREATMENT

There are two categories of treatment when treating PF: **passive** and **active** treatment. What does this mean?

When your body heals from a cut on your finger, is it passive or active? It's passive. Why? Because your body heals by itself naturally. Do you have to tell it to heal? No, it just does. You can give it things or do things to help speed up the healing, but it ultimately carries out the actual healing on its own. With regard to PF, this would be you, with your problem, simply giving your foot over, passively, to the doctor.

Passive **treatment** is when someone or something else does the work (for example, adjustments, orthotics, arch supports). It means you take a passive role and simply allow something or someone else, an outside source, to help fix the problem. Passive treatment is restricted neither to certain types of feet nor their associated problems. It refers to all treatments that are specific to a problem. A flat foot requires different treatment than does a high-arched foot. The doctor exposes your feet to passive treatments and lets them take care of the rest.

Active **treatment** is treatment in which *we* do the work. It's when you take an active role in your treatment: doing exercises, stretching, or resting your feet. *Active* treatment is specific to the type of problem as well.

Many cases can go unresolved or take a great length of time to heal when misapplication of these two types of treatment occurs relative to timing. Generally speaking, passive treatment should come first, allowing the structure and tissues to heal and restore function naturally before aggressive active therapies are incorporated. However, if passive treatment is not an option, active treatment is better than doing nothing at all. To obtain optimal results, applying both types of treatment is the best approach.

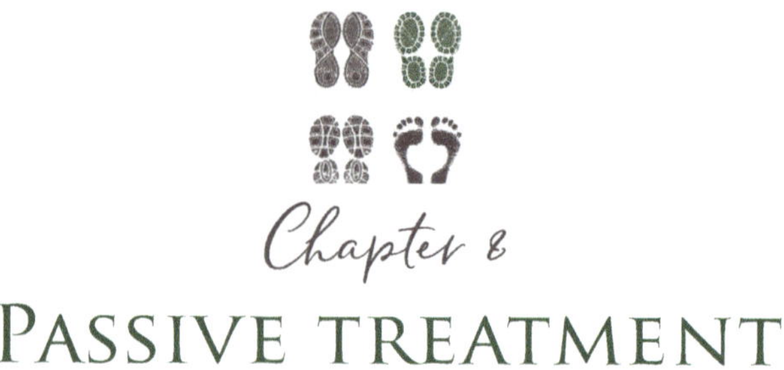

Chapter 8

PASSIVE TREATMENT

Scar tissue therapy

The first aspect of correcting any structural foot problem of a biomechanical nature is to assess the patient for tarsal subluxation. Why is this important? Because, as mentioned previously, we don't want inflexibility caused by locked bones/joints to lead to potential tissue damage. The way this tissue damage most often reveals itself is in the form of *scar tissue.*

Scar tissue is a byproduct of injured tissue. It can build up along and around the plantar fascia in plantar fasciitis patients. When scar tissue builds up it can be highly sensitive and very uncomfortable. It's also weaker in structural integrity, thus making it susceptible to further injury. It is important to break the scar tissue down in order to promote the healing process. This brings me to the first type of treatment that is applied, which is *scar tissue therapy*. It can be extremely effective for plantar fasciitis patients.

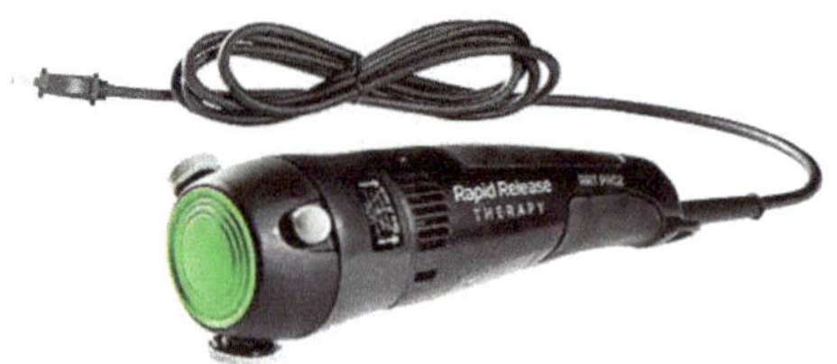

One of the ways that we approach this problem is by using devices that can be applied directly to the surface of the skin to break up the scar tissue passively. For this purpose, we use a vibrational frequency device that is highly effective; in fact, patients are even able to purchase such devices for home use. (See Rapid Release Therapy).

Adjustments

This is the most important of all passive treatments if subluxations exist in the patient's feet. The body, at times, is in a *guarded state*. This is the case when an individual is suffering from injured feet with subluxated tarsals, when the joints cannot release because of *abnormal muscle contraction , scar tissue build up, and displaced joint position.* Physiologically, *fast firing* is what's needed.

Fast firing is rapid input to the tissue that is so fast it resets and moves it effectively, sort of like popping something into place—and that's where chiropractic adjustment can be effective. In correlation with proper orthotics, adjustments can enhance movement to get the full effect with less discomfort.

Orthotics and supports

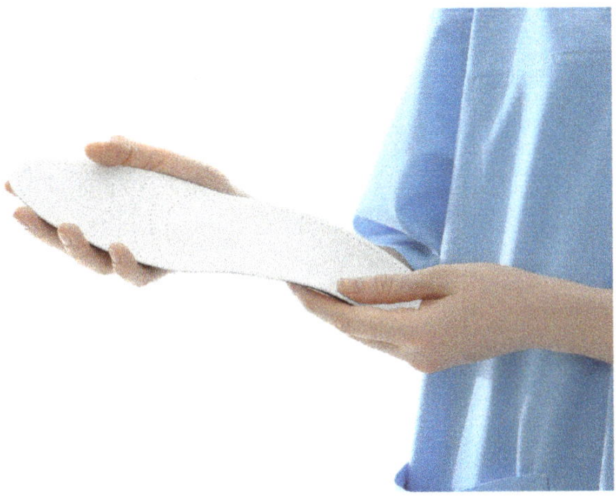

Orthotics can be one of the most effective treatment methods for plantar fasciitis. The key is timing. Placing a rigid orthotic on a locked joint can be counter-productive. Thus, the chiropractic approach is to adjust and realign the subluxated joints in the feet before implementing foot supports. Adjusting the feet first frees the tissues and allows greater flexibility and movement. The orthotic is then applied soon after to establish and support the changes. Thus, we want the locked joints to be freed up and *then* sustained for optimal results.

Each case is unique and might require either orthotics, inserts, arch supports, or heel cups, depending on the nature of the problem. The patients' needs vary with severity, age, and lifestyle.

Orthotics are usually custom-made and specifically tailored to the individual. They should be designed to realign, establish, and support the tissues of the feet. Podiatrists specialize in providing orthotics for various foot conditions and are an excellent source for the multiple types and brands available.

Functional orthotics tend to be more rigid and stiff, while *accommodative* orthotics are softer and more flexible.

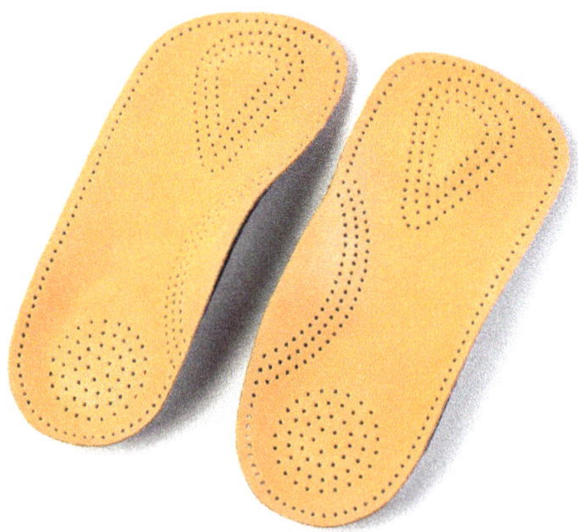

It's crucial that the orthotic is specific to the structural issue causing the symptoms.

Secondly, they should be worn with the proper shoes. Orthotics, inserts, and heel lifts should always correlate with the correct footwear in order to maximize optimal support. When footwear is poor-fitting or poorly designed, the orthotic can become more harmful than beneficial to the patient.

A growing concern over the years is that orthotics are often prescribed while the patient remains subluxated. This means the joints are "stuck" out of alignment. The orthotic, thus, tends to irritate the tissue, causing more discomfort as opposed to relief. Many patients have experienced "feeling worse" even after wearing expensive custom orthotics. As discussed previously, what frequently helps in these situations is mobilizing the locked joints first and then supporting them.

I have found that gel arch supports and the more flexible types of orthotics/inserts work very well with PF patients whose root cause is structural, that is, due to subluxations in the feet. These types of supports tend to mold to the foot more quickly and naturally while providing the needed support.

Generic shoe inserts can be purchased over the counter. These are great for added cushion and general support, but remember they are more of a "one-size-fits-all'. They are usually less effective for a foot deformity than a prescribed orthotic. However, they can be helpful for a normal or minimally irritated foot.

Each case is individual; thus, an overall understanding of the different types of support is crucial.

If self-prescribing, go back to the previous basics of foot pathologies to help determine what's needed.

Look at the diagram below:

FOOT ARCH TYPES

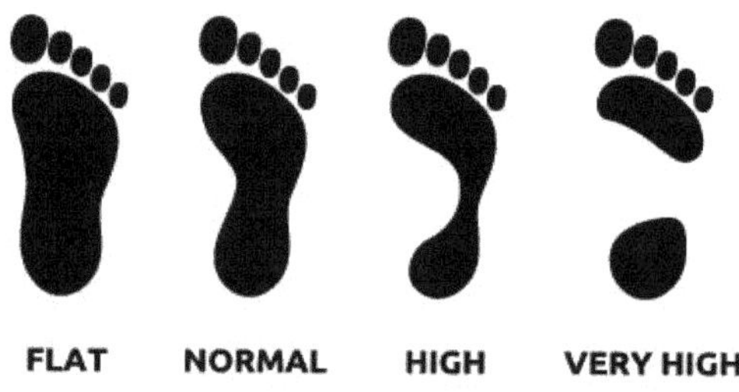

Once again, we see where pressure is placed on the bottom of each type of foot. So, getting the right insert is critical.

For example, for a *normal foot*, a standard insert providing a lot of cushioning and general support is the most effective. A person with a *flat foot* or *fallen arch* would wear one that provides plenty of arch support and helps to keep the foot and ankle from turning **inward** (pronation).

PLANOVALGUS FOOT

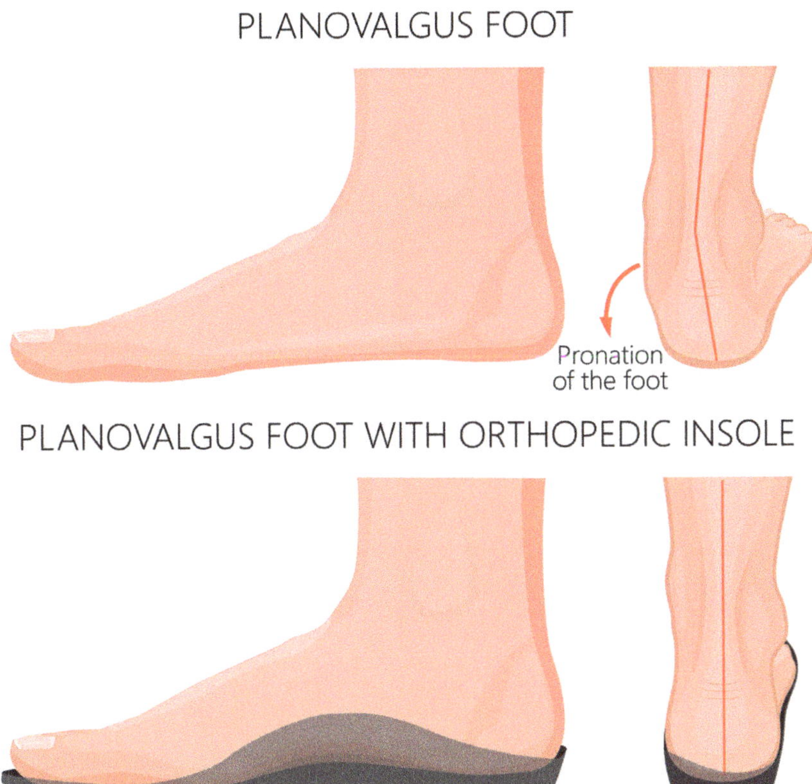

PLANOVALGUS FOOT WITH ORTHOPEDIC INSOLE

A *high-arched foot* would need one that has more heel and forefoot cushioning that, at the same time, provides lateral ankle support to help keep the feet from turning **outward (supination)**. This type of foot also tends to have *dropped metatarsals,* in particular the **second one**. Applying the correct orthotic or insert to address these issues specifically can be very effective in most cases.

Taping and wraps

Taping can be used as a means to support and stabilize feet; however, it's best to consult a healthcare professional on this as its effectiveness greatly depends on proper placement. Using stretch tape generally works best. The one drawback with taping is that it can potentially affect the skin in some cases (causing breakouts, blisters, etc.).

We won't discuss specific techniques at this time, but just be aware that taping would be considered a possibility in the category of passive treatment. The individual could use therapy/body tape to hold the bones or joints in a supported position.

Stretching (Being stretched)

Passive stretching would involve the doctor or therapist stretching your foot for you. This type of stretching would be up to the practitioner based on the patient's condition.

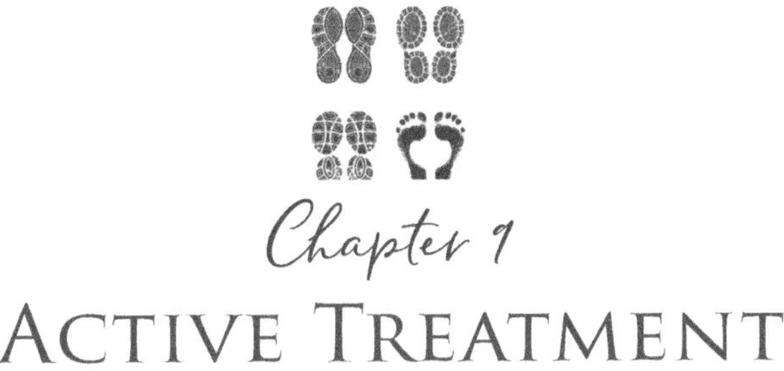

Chapter 9

ACTIVE TREATMENT

Active treatment is where you, for the most part, do the majority of the work, sometimes with and sometimes without a device.

Remember this: **if active treatment causes more discomfort, STOP!**

If you can't go see your doctor right away, there are some things you can do to help yourself. The first thing that you can do, if you haven't already, is to consult me, a podiatrist, or your doctor to find out if you have the right footwear (more on that to come).

Secondly, what type of structural issues do you think you may have? Do you have a flat foot? Do you have a high-arched foot? If so, do you have an orthotic? And what type of orthotic do you have? If you don't, have you tried one? Secondly, does it feel like your foot is rigid and stuck? If so, you may have subluxations in your feet. Third, what stretches have you done? What stretches do you know? If you have flat feet, there are specific types of stretches you can do. If you have high-arched feet, there are specific stretches you can do for them as well. Do you run? If you run, have you been checked for stress fractures? And, what types of running shoes are you using? How much cushioning do you have in the shoes? These are all questions to ask yourself before active treatment and prior to seeing your doctor.

Stretching

The best times to do active stretching are in the morning and before exercising. Starting the day with a good stretch routine helps our bodies to efficiently handle the load of everyday life that can cause stress to our skeletal structure. Maintaining flexibility in our muscles and joints is vital to overall structural health and should be a part of any regular fitness routine.

Towel or grab stretch

While seated on the floor, put your leg out in front of you. Take a towel or cloth and wrap it around the ball of your foot (you can also just grab the ball of your foot with your hand); one foot at a time actually works best for remaining in a comfortable, relaxed position. Pull your foot back toward your shin and hold the stretch for one minute. Do each foot three times.

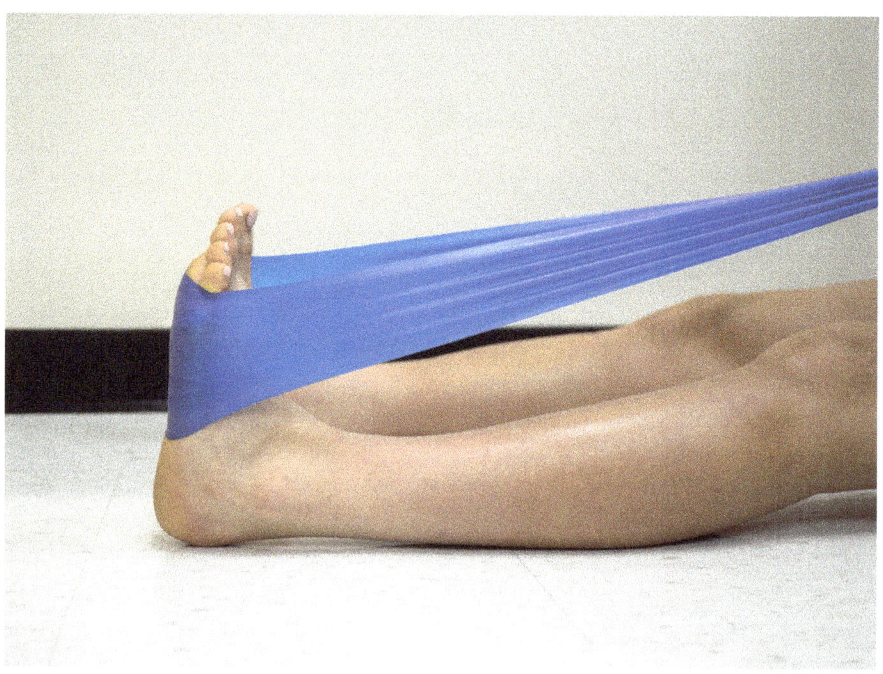

Calf/ankle stretch

Place your hands against the wall and place one foot back (the farther back it goes, the deeper the stretch). Stay within your own limitations, but lock your leg and slowly lower your heel to the ground until your foot is flat. Hold that stretch for 60 seconds.

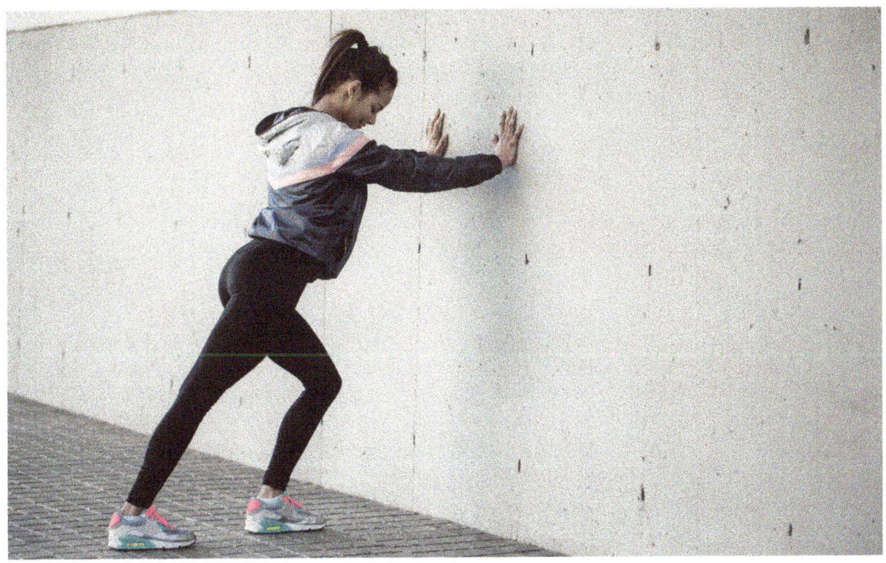

Yoga Toes

Yoga toes are small plastic devices that allow a fantastic stretch between the toes. They are easy to use and can really relax the foot muscles. They can generally be found to purchase online and typically range anywhere from $15-$40.

Stair stretch

This is similar to the calf stretch, except with a stair or small step. With your heel on the ground, place the ball of your foot on the edge of a small step or against a wall. Lean forward in a similar way as the calf stretch until you feel the stretch in the calf and foot. Using this method is more intense, with a deeper stretch, so you will feel the stretch sooner without having to lean forward as much.

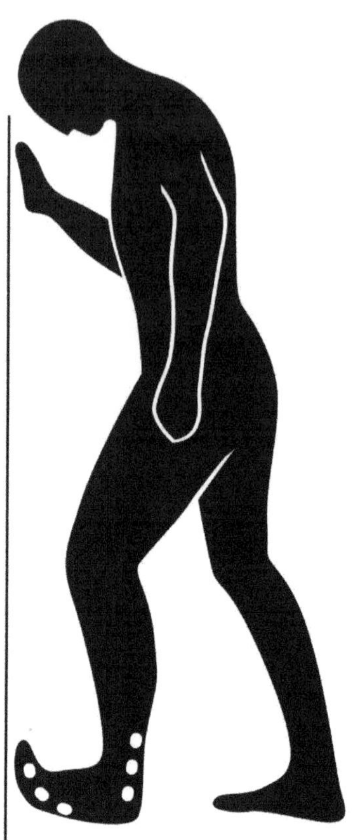

Exercises

Exercises for the feet will be a little more specific to the type of foot problem involved because some muscles will be weak in one type of problem, whereas the same muscles will be strong in another type of foot problem. Exercises can be done for rehabilitation but also with healthy feet for prevention and overall strength.

In this section, we will talk about which ones apply to which conditions. To start with, again, these are very general, and your healthcare practitioner or physical therapist may add or subtract from these, depending on your condition.

Flat Feet or Normal Foot Shape with Associated PF

Flat feet exercises

Flat feet involve bones that have been shifted inward and downward on the inner part of the arch. The two main bones that shift are the *navicular* bone and the *medial cuneiform* bone. Because they shift downward and inward, proper arch support and proper footwear are of the utmost importance. The goal is to shift the arch back into its proper position. With this condition, we want to implement exercises that are going to strengthen the muscles of the inner arch and ankle, thereby creating flexibility in motion.

Toe curls

The first exercise is known as *toe curls*. In a seated position, we simply point the toes down and try to curl them as far underneath our feet as we can.

In other words, imagine touching your toes to your heel. Hold that flexed position for at least 30 seconds. Do three sets of three curls on each foot. This can also be done with a towel.

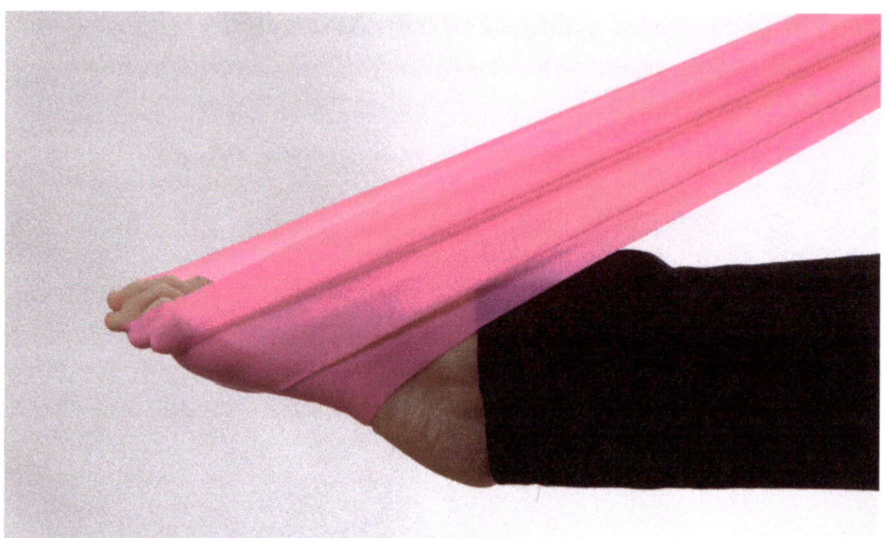

Ankle circles

The second exercise we implement is ankle circles. These are tremendous for developing both strength and flexibilty at the same time. Circle the foot inward and clockwise eight times; then, circle it outward and counterclockwise eight times. Do three sets of inward and outward curls with each foot.

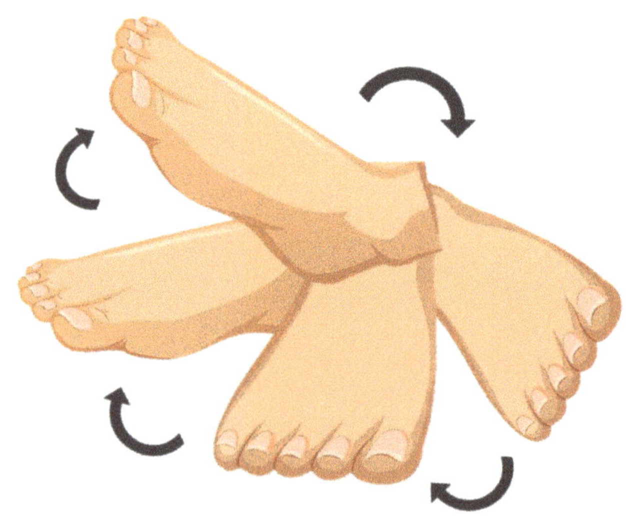

Toe lifting

Grab a marble, pencil, or other small object (one that won't cut your skin) with your toes and lift your foot off the floor, except for your heel. Keep your heel touching the floor. Hold the object for five seconds while curling your arch at the same time.

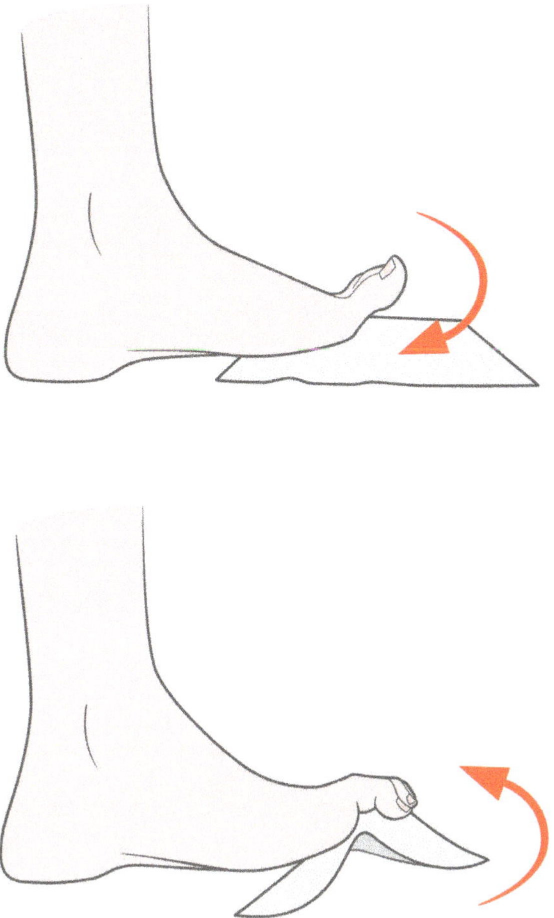

Lower your foot back down to the floor and release. Repeat this five times. If your leg cramps during this exercise, stop and do two sets of ankle circles and stair stretches, then try this again when you feel comfortable enough to do so.

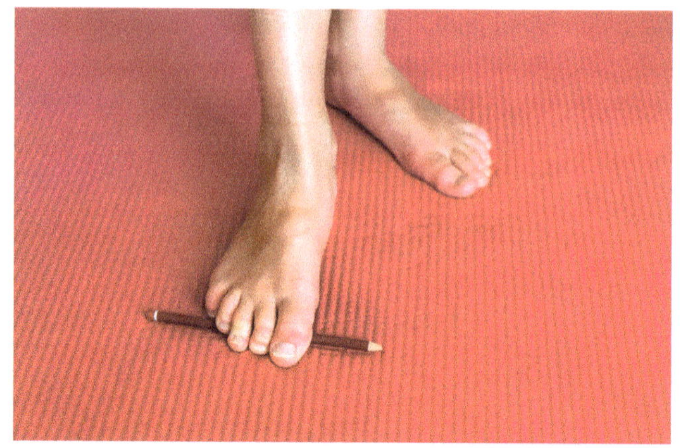

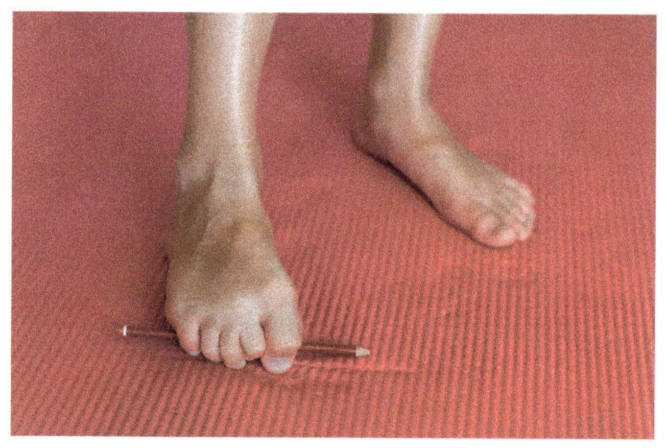

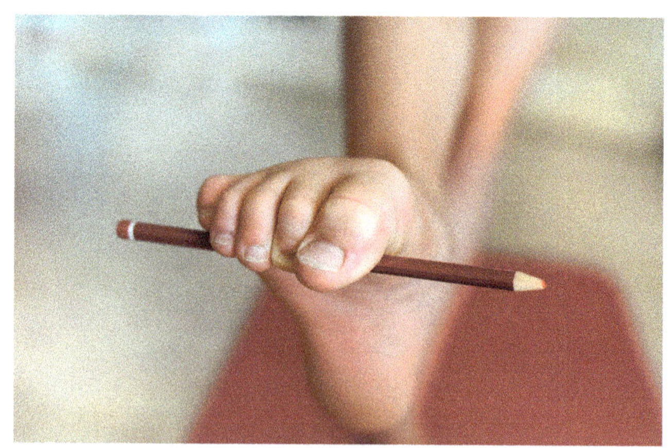

Sand walking

If you live near a beach or any place that has sand, walking in sand barefoot is tremendously beneficial for your feet. It allows simultaneous stretching and contraction of different foot muscles with every step. If you do not live near the ocean, you can use a sandbox. Either way, walking in sand helps to stretch in between the joints gently. It helps to get everything moving in a very natural way and to open things up; joints get a lot of their nourishment through motion.

High-Arched Foot exercises

Pulling your toes up toward your shin

In a comfortable, seated position with your legs flat out in front of you or just hanging down from a chair, pull your toes back toward your shin. Imagine trying to touch your shin bone. Hold this position for 60 seconds and repeat it five times with each foot. This exercise is excellent for women who wear heels quite frequently.

Ankle circles

Most individuals with this type of foot have lateral (outside part) ankle instability.

These are the same circles we described earlier. Those with high arches should do eight outward circles and four inward circles per set. Repeat this 10 times for each foot.

Sand walking

The same applies to high arches as it does to flat arches in terms of walking in sand.

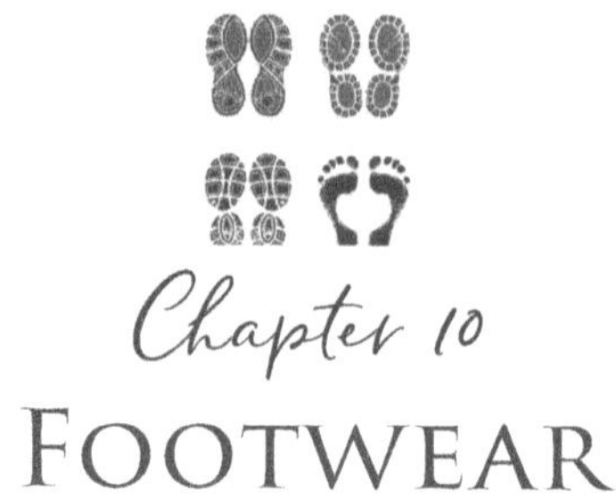

Chapter 10

FOOTWEAR

Of all the chapters of this book, this one has the most significant impact on recovery. Footwear can have a tremendous effect on the structure of our feet. In today's culture, people often wear different types of shoes based on how they look rather than how they feel. We seem to base our decisions many times on fashion and what's "in" as opposed to what's best. As a result, many women wear high heels excessively.

For example, if I were to wear a shoe that was very narrow in the toe area, that would not allow my toes to expand. Over time, the tissues that surround the muscles near the front of my foot would start to deform and weaken because they would not be allowed to function properly. This could lead to a cascade of problems, creating a domino effect that could lead to PF.

So, why is it important to find proper footwear? It's important because we want to avoid chronic issues that cannot be corrected later on in life.

How do we know what to wear? What footwear is appropriate? Before shoes existed, many people went barefoot or wore sandals. I would venture to say there was very little constriction on their feet back then. We weren't designed to have major constriction around our joints. The key to a good shoe is whether it allows for the natural movement of the joints in our feet.

One of the healthiest ways to allow the joints of our feet to move freely and open up is sand walking, as previously mentioned. This is a very healthy way to stretch the ligaments, tendons, and muscles in the feet. What we put on our feet should mimic this same natural motion, in which all the joints are free to move. Your shoes must fit properly; they must neither be too tight, too small, nor too big in order for this to happen. And, based on the structure of your foot, the shoes should fit properly in conjunction with compensating for any existing abnormalities.

There is also another element of shoes that many of us are not familiar with, although it can play a major role in the health of our feet. It's the actual *geometrical shape* of the shoe, or what's called the *last*.

The last is the mold the shoe manufacturer uses to form the actual shoe. It is one of the most important general components of the shoe; it can greatly affect the structure of our feet.

The key here is the *shape of the bottom of the last*. The shaped mold used in the configuration of the bottom of your shoe actually determines how well you function mechanically.

The last can be **straight** from heel to toe, **curved** like a banana heel to toe, or just in between the two extremes, which is called a **standard** last.

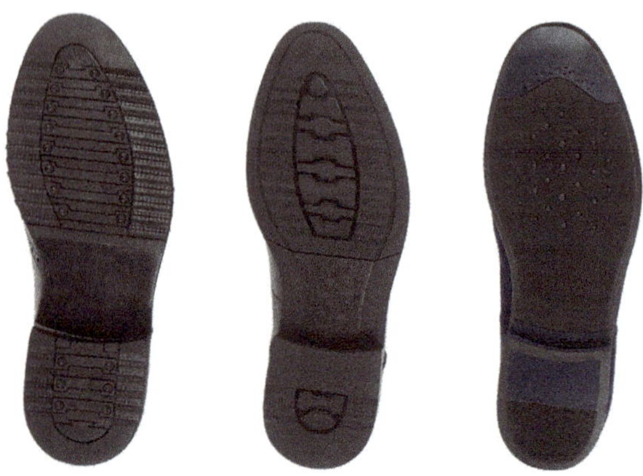

The force and pressure that are applied to the bottom of each foot type will be different in certain areas—more in some and less in others.

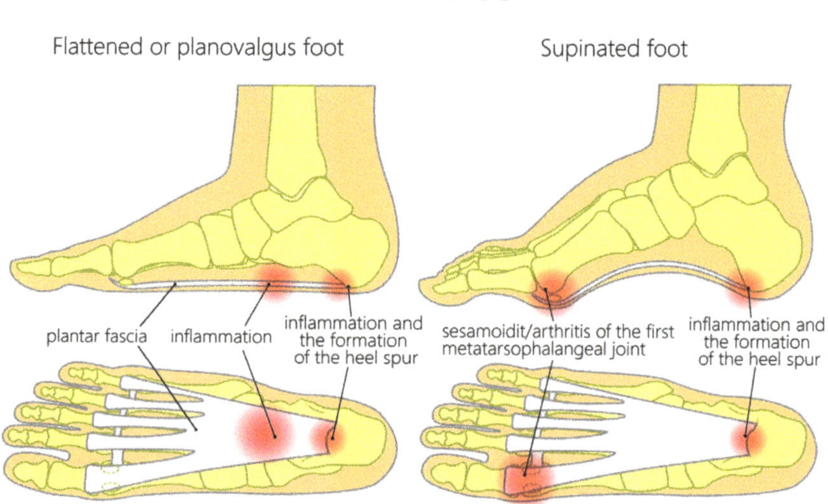

Knowing how to match the type of foot with the correctly shaped bottom of the shoe will enhance your feet mechanically as opposed to making them worse over time.

Finding shoes that help with pronation (inward rolling of the foot and/or ankle) and supination (outward rolling of foot and/or ankle) can make a tremendous difference in keeping the foot mechanics working properly.

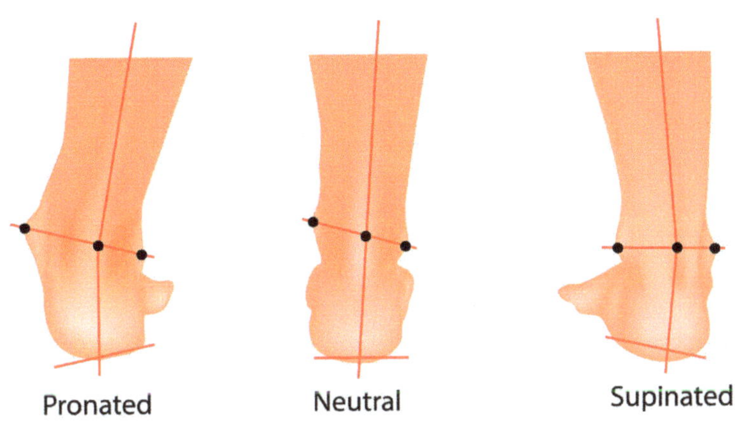

Diagram of right foot from behind. From right to left: pronated, normal, and supinated weight-bearing

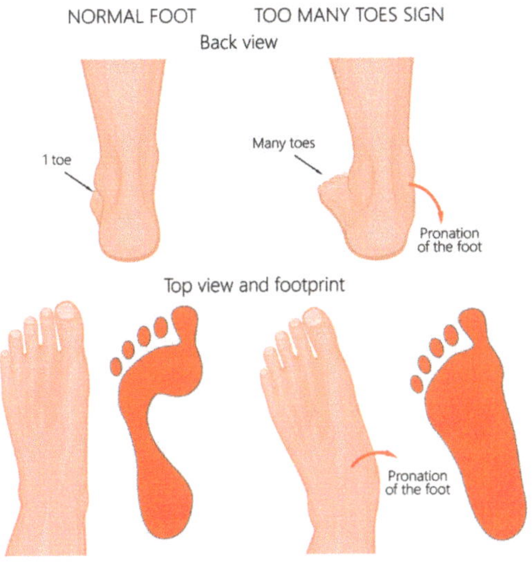

Shoe last for flat feet

Flat feet are often accompanied by something called *pronation*. Pronation is an inward rolling of the ankle. This can put tremendous pressure on the inside portion of the arch and ankle while standing or walking. Over time, this is a lot of wear and tear and stress to the fascia.

What we want is a *motion control* shoe. This is especially important when a runner, walker or hiker has flat feet.

These shoes offer the benefit of keeping the ankle from rolling inward too much while it is pounding against the ground. Without the right support, this can lead not only to PF but also to ankle, knee, hip, and back problems. Therefore, the type of shoe people with flat feet should use is a ***straight lasted* shoe.**

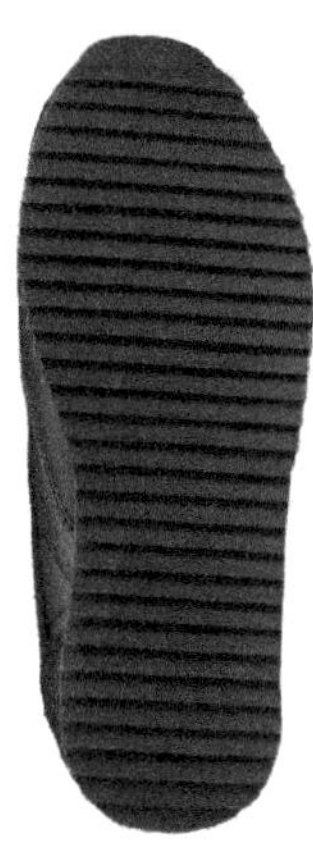

Shoes for high-arched feet

The main areas of consideration here are the *instep* and *supination*. Generally, an individual with high-arched feet needs a shoe that will accommodate a high instep. It's important to make sure there is plenty of space. Also, this particular type of foot has the tendency to sometimes *supinate* (outward rolling of the foot and ankle when walking).

The best type of shoe for this type of foot has a *curved last*. This will help the foot roll back inward when walking or running. In the picture of the sole of a curved-last shoe, notice that in comparison to a straight line, the shape is more like that of a banana.

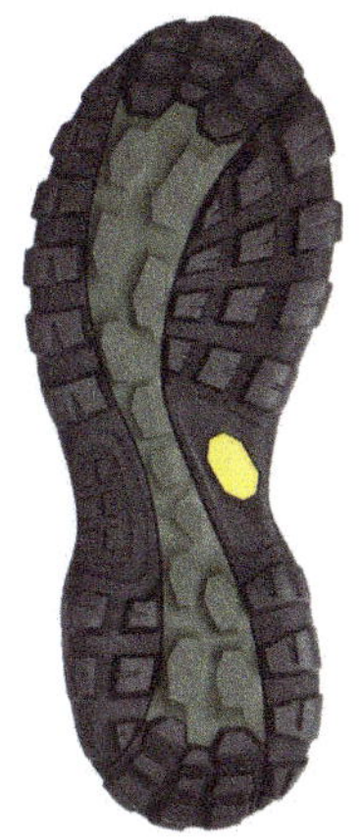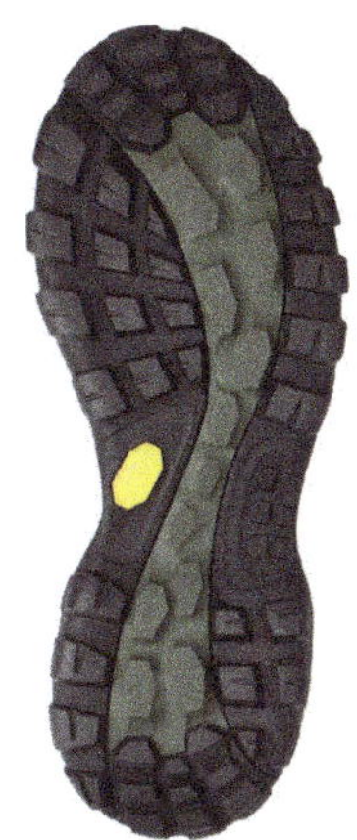

Cushioning

Cushioning is extremely important in helping to recover from PF. Wearing well-cushioned shoes (especially in the morning on hard surfaces) can help PF injuries heal and recover more quickly and thoroughly. There are several brands out there that have great cushioned soles. Take the time to try and find what feels and fits best. The brand we highly recommend in the clinic is **MBT**. MBT stands for ***Masai Barefoot Technology***. The superior design of this shoe provides cushion and support, while helping to establish proper foot mechanics and gate cycle. As the name implies, they mimic barefoot walking on natural terrain. Barefoot walking in the sand, as previously mentioned, can be very beneficial.

Running shoes

Having the correct type of running shoe is very important as the force of impact during running is significantly more when compared to walking. It is especially critical for high-mileage runners who run several miles per day as part of their standard routine.

Running can have an adverse effect on the joints of the body over time. Having the proper equipment is extremely important. Specifically, the type of surface determines several factors of the impact. Thus, running on hard surfaces requires more cushioning and protection.

For example, if someone is doing high-mileage running on asphalt, concrete, or other hard surfaces, they're going to need much more cushioning in their shoes to absorb the shock going into the joints.

If an individual is running on hills, a different type of impact force is in play. Furthermore, the force of impact while running uphill can be different than running downhill because the stride is slightly different.

One way to help absorb some of the impact when running downhill is to imagine running on one's heels. It actually helps to center, innately and biomechanically, the placement of the foot during the stride. In this way, it can reduce stress on the joints.

For a runner, the principles of the most appropriately shaped shoe for certain foot types are even more applicable. As mentioned earlier, a straight lasted shoe is better for a pronator than is a curved lasted shoe as the former supports the inner part of the ankle when walking or running. There are certain types that have roller bars built into the inside portion of the midsole. The material is denser and designed to provide extra support. The curved lasted shoe is obviously better for a high-arched supinator when striking the ground.

Many times, when people are fitted at a running shoe store, they run on a computerized treadmill. However, it is important to keep in mind that this doesn't identify foot-type deformities. If necessary, refer back to previous chapters in this book to help you with your purchase decision.

There are a great many brands out there. Make your choice based on what's best for your foot type first, not by the brand. Thus, the most important step in finding out which brand works for you is to find out whether you have a flat or high-arched foot and to understand what that means. Once you have identified your type, try on several pairs as each brand and shoe type will have different variations that may have profound effects on performance.

High heels

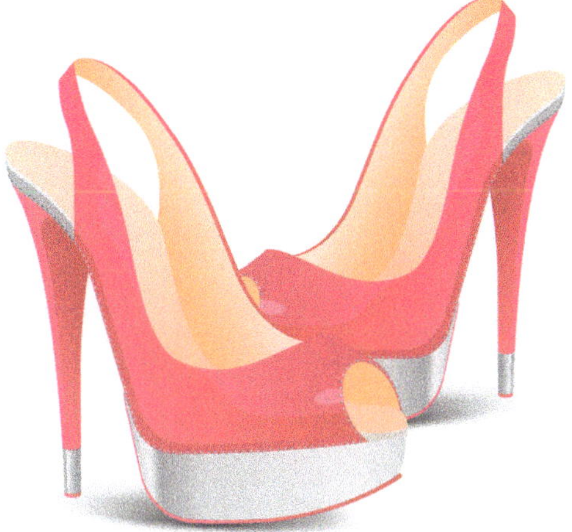

Some women may not like what I'm about to say regarding high heels, but this is a book about helping to prevent plantar fasciitis; unfortunately, high heels can potentially do tremendous damage to the foot.

The human foot was not made to walk on its toes constantly. When wearing heels, the foot is in a downward flexed position, changing the dynamics of normal weightbearing when standing or walking. Over time, this can put tremendous stress on the supporting tissues in the feet, increasing the risk of injury.

Case in point: a patient of mine came in on crutches. The mechanism that caused the onset of her injury was that she was chasing her kid down the sidewalk in high heels. As a result, her foot was seriously injured.

In terms of foot positioning, when wearing high heels, essentially, the wearer is walking on the balls of the feet, sometimes for hours each day.

This, in turn, can initiate a cascading-domino effect that creates problems in the hips, knees, and back. It also creates the potential for bunions and other issues that may or may not be directly related to plantar fasciitis.

Approximately 72% of women will wear high heels in their lifetime. It's the ultimate sacrifice of foot pain for fashion, but it isn't just foot pain that is the issue. It's the other issues that affect the body. It's problems such as arthritis, anatomical deformities, joint pain, and inflammation. The posture can be adversely affected due to the overall imbalance caused by heels for the center of gravity of the body **(see Figure A).**

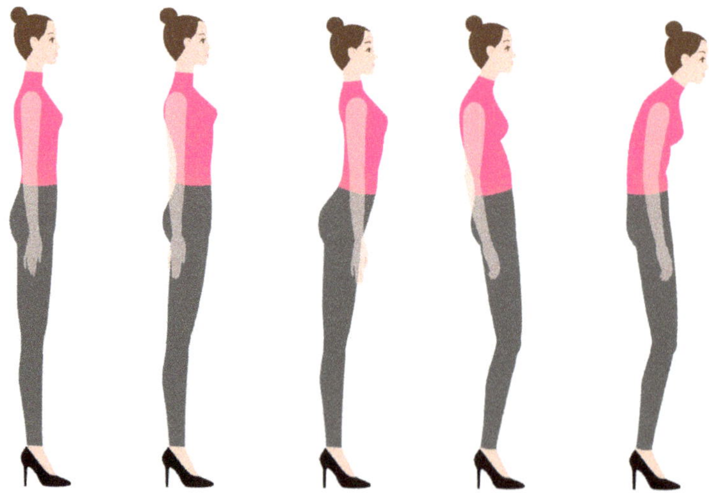

Figure A) The effects of heels over time on posture.

In the figure, we see that the head ends up in a forward position out in front of the rib cage, causing imbalance throughout the rest of the skeletal system.

These are some of the adverse effects that can be caused by the excessive use of high heels:

1. Tremendous pressure on the ball of the foot

How high the heel is determines the amount of pressure on the forefoot. A four-inch heel results in more pressure on the balls of the feet than does a two-inch heel. This pressure can eventually lead to problems in the Achilles tendon and calf. The muscles and tendons can become extremely tight over time, increasing the risk of further injury. Wearing high heels can also lead to bunions, corns, and hammertoes.

2. Knee pain

Excessive pressure on the balls of the feet can cause extra pressure on the knee joints. This can lead to knee problems, discomfort, chronic knee pain, and difficulty walking.

3. Anterior pelvic tilt

This condition can cause increased arching of the lower back. The body has to compensate for the amount of elevation of the foot and heels and the pressure on the forefoot. In order to keep the body balanced, the hips and back tend to push forward. What this can do is cause back and pelvic misalignments, which can lead to pinched nerves, tightened muscles, and lower back pain.

4. Poor posture

Wearing heels mimics walking up a ramp; when the heels are taken off, the body has to adapt. As a result, it can be very difficult for the body to shift back and forth between the two postures as it attempts to keep the body balanced. In other words, when a person becomes adapted to walking on their toes, the body will start to reposition in such a way that it adapts to keeping the individual balanced in that posture. Once the shoes are taken off, however, the body has to readapt to keep everything balanced. Muscles and ligaments can become deformed over time in such a way that the posture can be altered even when not wearing heels. This can create further issues, such as arthritis, injured muscles, and discomfort.

5. Neuromas, hammertoes, dropped metatarsals

If high heels are 3-4 inches high and have pointy toes (or a pointy toe box), this can squeeze the toes together in such a way that it can increase the pressure on a nerve, causing it to expand and create what's called a *neuroma*. It can cause calluses, along with built-up calcification on the metatarsals.

6. Cavus foot or high arch

Because the foot is placed in a position as if the individual is standing on their toes, once the shoes come off, the metatarsals can appear to be dropped; as such, the arch will follow, creating a high-arched type of foot. This can then cause tightness in the Achilles tendon and calf, subsequently causing areas of the foot to become painful, such as the heel or forefoot. Over time, this tends to end in PF.

7. Achilles tendon rupture

Constant tightening of the Achilles tendon and calf muscles can create a weakening of the proteins in the cartilage and connective tissue of the Achilles tendon. This can make it susceptible to possible rupture, even without a traumatic event. That's why if an individual is going to wear heels on a regular basis, it is very important to stretch.

Suggestions

Some solutions to help protect the feet from damage caused by the prolonged wearing of heels are as follows:

- Regular stretching is important to do on a daily basis, either with or without heels. One stretch that can be done is to find a one-inch block, book, or step and place the forefoot on the edge of it. Then, lean forward at the waist and try to touch your toe, stretching the back of the calf and the ankle. Do one leg at a time and try to hold the position for 30-45 seconds. This can help to keep the calf loose and the Achilles tendon from overtightening.

- Wear heels in moderation. Perhaps limit how often and how long you wear them. Save them for special occasions or only wear them when necessary for work.

- Put on recovery shoes immediately after wearing them. Comfortable cushioned shoes after a few hours of heels can go a long way. Giving your feet a break helps them to recover more quickly.

- A good foot massage after a long day in heels can be heaven for the feet. There are mechanical foot therapy machines available now that can give a pretty good massage depending on the model.

- Stretch daily. Stretching is vital to preventing injuries. As mentioned previously, this cannot be overemphasized. Stretch the entire body. *Yoga* is a fantastic method to develop overall flexibilty and strength. Regular stretching of the calf and Achilles tendon can help offset overall tightness caused by the excessive use of heels.

- Get rid of them! Notice how I suggested this one last? Lol. I realize that this is unlikely. In reality, they are often required for work and business, as well as special occasions. However, if it is possible to do so, it is something to ponder after weighing the health benefits.

It's in our nature and DNA to walk correctly. As I mentioned earlier, one of the healthiest things and one of the exercises I prescribe to my PF patients is walking in sand. If you really want to know your natural gait cycle, walk in sand. If our feet mimic this in our shoes, we've got a winner! This means that the joints aren't constricted and are free to move. All this should be achieved, however, without the shoes being too big. Thus, emphasizing once again the importance of proper fitting footwear that is specific to your foot type.

Remember, it starts with *our feet.* The issue is not so much just walking properly—it's having feet that are ready and able to do so. We are adaptive creatures: We're adaptive to our environment, and we're adaptive to our structure. We're adaptive in the sense that we don't want to feel discomfort, and we don't want to feel pain. We consciously and subconsciously adapt our bodies to ensure that our daily lives will not cause discomfort. At the same time, if our shoes are wrong, we sometimes overlook this principle for the sake of fashion. As a result, the tissue in our feet becomes damaged. Thus, make sure out of all the sections in this book, this one really hits home. Weigh the consequences carefully when choosing what to put on your feet. We can sometimes assume that a shoe works if it fits our fashion style. Be sure to examine the fit and performance first and, most importantly, whether it's right for your foot type.

CONCLUSION

Throughout over two decades of clinical practice, I have seen case after case of patients who come in with structural issues stemming from root causes that they don't even know exist.

Once they adopt the structural and mechanical changes necessary, I see tremendous recoveries, tremendous relief, and people leaving with healthy, happy feet.

I've seen it experientially. Therefore, my thoughts are that one should not be too quick to undergo a surgical procedure, nor be too quick just to give up and take steroid injections, nor accept defeat.

If something can be done naturally, try that first. The best medicine cabinet that God has given us in the world today is the medicine cabinet that's within our own body.

As mentioned, in the Psalm, it says our bodies *are fearfully and wonderfully made.* One of the greatest gifts that God gave us is our body's ability to self-heal—the ability to heal naturally. When all of the healing components are activated, it is more powerful than any drug or anything else that man can make.

My hope and prayer is that all the PF sufferers reading this book will take something from this material and immediately apply it in such a way that it makes a healthy, positive difference.

God Bless!

BIBLIOGRAPHY

"Amount of Water in the Human Body." Nestlé Waters. Accessed March 16, 2020. https://www.nestle-waters.com/learn-about-water/general-needs/how-much-water-is-in-the-human-body.

"Analysis of Data on the Prevalence and Pharmacologic Treatment of Plantar Fasciitis Pain." National Center for Complementary and Integrative Health. U.S. Department of Health and Human Services, July 25, 2018. https://nccih.nih.gov/research/results/spotlight/Plantar-Fasciitis-Pain.

Andersen, Jens Jakob. "Marathon Statistics 2019 Worldwide (Research)." Athletic shoe reviews, June 20, 1970. https://runrepeat.com/research-marathon-performance-across-nations.

"Are Steroid Injections Safe for Plantar Fasciitis and Heel Pain?" Heel That Pain. Accessed March 16, 2020. https://heelthatpain.com/plantar-fasciitis/corticosteroid-injections/.

Baravarian, Bob. "Rethinking The Treatment Options For Plantar Fasciitis." Podiatry Today, March 14, 2019. https://www.podiatrytoday.com/rethinking-treatment-options-plantar-fasciitis.

Cross, Rod. "Standing, Walking, Running, and Jumping on a Force Plate." Accessed March 1, 2020. http://www.physics.usyd.edu.au/~cross/PUBLICATIONS/6. StandingForcePlate.PDF.

"Cuboid Syndrome." Wikipedia. Wikimedia Foundation, November 30, 2019. https://en.wikipedia.org/wiki/Cuboid_syndrome.

Dresden, Danielle. "Cuboid Syndrome: What It Is, Treatment, and Recovery." Medical News Today. MediLexicon International, April 26, 2018. https://www.medicalnewstoday.com/articles/321626.

Durall, Chris J. "Examination and Treatment of Cuboid Syndrome: a Literature Review." Sports health. SAGE Publications, November 2011. https://www.ncbi.nlm.nih.gov/pmc/articles/PMC3445231/.

Foot, The Athlete's. "Your Feet on Running vs. Your Feet on Walking." Mashable. Mashable, June 14, 2016. https://mashable.com/2016/06/13/running-vs-walking/.

"How High Heels Affect Your Body." Spine Health Institute. Accessed March 16, 2020. http://www.thespinehealthinstitute.com/news-room/health-blog/how-high-heels-affect-your-body.

"How Stress Affects Your Body and Behavior." Mayo Clinic. Mayo Foundation for Medical Education and Research, April 4, 2019. https://www.mayoclinic.org/healthy-lifestyle/stress-management/in-depth/stress-symptoms/art-20050987.

Human Movement Sciences. "Impact Forces of Walking and Running at the Same Intensity : The Journal of Strength & Conditioning Research." LWW. Accessed March 16, 2020. https://journals.lww.com/nsca-jscr/fulltext/2016/04000/impact_forces_of_walking_and_running_at_the_same.19.aspx.

"Issaquah Podiatrists Providing the Most Complete Foot & Ankle Treatment to The Eastside." Issaquah Foot & Ankle Specialists. Accessed March 16, 2020. https://www.bestfootdoc.com/faqs/all-about-cortisone-injections-for-plantar-fasciitis.cfm.

"Last." Wikipedia. Wikimedia Foundation, March 6, 2020. https://en.wikipedia.org/wiki/Last.

McCoy, ByKrisha, Joseph Bennington-Castro, Lynn Marks, Diana Rodriguez, and Jennifer Acosta Scott. "8 Foot Exercises for Bunions: Everyday Health." EverydayHealth.com. Accessed March 16, 2020. https://www.everydayhealth.com/foot-health/8-foot-exercises-for-bunions.aspx.

Minnis DPT, Gregory. "Everything You Need to Know About Heel Spurs." Healthline. Accessed November 22, 2019. https://www.healthline.com/health/heel-spurs.

Minnis DPT, Gregory. "Exercises for Flat Feet." Healthline, October 16, 2018. https://www.healthline.com/health/flat-feet-exercises.

Minnis DPT, Gregory. "Orthotics: Are They the Answer to Your Foot, Leg, or Back Pain?" Healthline, March 19, 2019. https://www.healthline.com/health/bone-health/orthotics.

myPhysioSA. "Best Physio Exercises to Help Flat Feet." myPhysioSA. myPhysioSA, January 30, 2020. https://myphysiosa.com.au/best-physio-exercises-to-help-flat-feet-by-mount-barker-adelaide-physiotherapist-david/.

"Office of Dietary Supplements - Vitamin C." NIH Office of Dietary Supplements. U.S. Department of Health and Human Services. Accessed March 16, 2020. https://ods.od.nih.gov/factsheets/VitaminC-HealthProfessional/#h1.

"Orthotic Management of the Pes Cavus Foot." Lower Extremity Review Magazine. Accessed March 16, 2020. https://lermagazine.com/article/orthotic-management-of-the-pes-cavus-foot.

Palomo-López, Patricia, Ricardo Becerro-de-Bengoa-Vallejo, Marta Elena Losa-Iglesias, David Rodríguez-Sanz, César Calvo-Lobo, and Daniel López-López. "Impact of Plantar Fasciitis on the Quality of Life of Male and Female: JPR."

Journal of Pain Research. Dove Press, April 27, 2018. https://
www.dovepress.com/impact-of-plantar-fasciitis-on-the-quality-
of-life-of-male-and-female--peer-reviewed-fulltext-article-JPR.

Praderio, Caroline. "I Wore High Heels to Work for Two Weeks
Straight and Was Shocked by What It Did to My Body."
Insider. Insider, May 22, 2017. https://www.insider.com/
wearing-heels-every-day-risks-2017-5.

Quench USA, Inc. "Nearly 80 Percent Of Working Americans
Say They Don't Drink Enough Water: Quench Survey." PR
Newswire: press release distribution, targeting, monitoring and
marketing, June 27, 2018. https://www.prnewswire.com/news-
releases/nearly-80-percent-of-working-americans-say-they-
dont-drink-enough-water-quench-survey-300668537.html.

"Running Barefoot or in Minimal Footwear." Running Barefoot:
Home. Accessed March 16, 2020. http://barefootrunning.fas.
harvard.edu/4BiomechanicsofFootStrike.html.

Schumacker, Lauren. "7 Scary Things That Can
Happen When You Wear Heels Too Much."
Insider, May 3, 2018. https://www.insider.com/
things-that-happen-to-feet-when-you-wear-heels-2018-5.

Searing, Linda. "The Big Number: 2 Million Americans Get Treated
for Heel Pain Caused by Plantar Fasciitis." The Washington Post.
WP Company, November 25, 2019. https://www.washingtonpost.
com/health/the-big-number-2-million-americans-get-treated-for-
heel-pain-caused-by-plantar-fasciitis/2019/11/22/0dfe89e8-0c7a-
11ea-97ac-a7ccc8dd1ebc_story.html.

Team, Joint. "7 Ways to Ease Bunion Pain Without Surgery."
Health Essentials from Cleveland Clinic. Health Essentials from
Cleveland Clinic, October 11, 2019. https://health.clevelandclinic.
org/7-ways-to-ease-your-bunions-without-surgery/.

Tongen, Anthony E, and Roshna E Wunderlich. "Biomechanics of Running and Walking." In Biomechanics of Running and Walking, 1–12. Accessed March 2020. http://www.mathaware. org/mam/2010/essays/TongenWunderlichRunWalk.pdf.

"Types of Orthotics." Foot & Ankle Institute - Foot Doctor Saint George, UT 84770, Hurricane, UT 84737, Cedar City, UT 84720 and Mesquite, NV 89027, also serving Beaver and Panguitch. Accessed March 16, 2020. https://www.feetnet.com/ blog/item/184-types-of-orthotics.html.

Wheeler, Tyler. "Knee Pain & Injuries: Causes, Treatment, & Prevention." WebMD. WebMD, September 13, 2019. https://www.webmd.com/pain-management/knee-pain/ knee-pain-causes.

Chicago Manual of Style 16th edition (full note) formatting by CitationMachine.net.